To Live Each Moment

One Woman's Struggle Against Cancer

Janet Britton

InterVarsity Press
Downers Grove
Illinois 60515

InterVarsity Press is the book-publishing division of Inter-Varsity Christian Fellowship, a student movement active on campus at hundreds of universities, colleges and schools of nursing. For information about local and regional activities, write IVCF, 233 Langdon St., Madison, WI 53703.

Distributed in Canada through InterVarsity Press, 860 Denison St., Unit 3, Markham, Ontario L3R 4H1, Canada.

Cover photograph (not the author): David Singer

ISBN 0-87784-282-5

Printed in the United States of America

Library of Congress Cataloging in Publication Data

Britton, Janet, 1947-
    To live each moment.

    1. Britton, Janet, 1947- .   2. Breast—Cancer—
Patients—United States—Biography.   3. Christian life—
1960-   .   I. Title.
RC280.B8B74   1984   362.1'96994'0924 [B]   83-26532
ISBN 0-87784-282-5

20 19 18 17 16 15 14 13 12 11 10 9 8 7 6 5 4 3 2 1

99 98 97 96 95 94 93 92 91 90 89 88 87 86 85 84

Let Me Explain...

Raggedy Anns, needlepoint wall hangings, quilts and afghans —your friends' mothers create treasures for their children. I've never enjoyed working on projects of thread and yarn. So for you, my little ones, I've created a gift of words, the material I weave most comfortably.

Your dad and I have always tried to deal openly with words— even ones some people view shocking. We believe when important topics are avoided, facts and emotions get jumbled; misinformation and confusion result. That's why we've discussed that word *cancer* with you both—the details of treatment, our reactions, our fears.

I've used words to explain my impressions of my illness; I think dealing with words is important. But I want you both to always try to see behind the words people use. Remember how I'm calm when I want to scream and how Daddy screams when he wants to cry. Sometimes the most important words are the ones *not* spoken. Listen to hear the anger behind the smile—the tears behind the laughter.

This gift of words is like the afghans that your friends' mothers make. One strand of yarn doesn't look like much. But when we step back and view the completed project, we can see the beauty of the pattern that results from the weaving of individual strands together. My afghan to you was knit from the strands of individual lives—those of our family; of members of the medical community, the church and my school; and of friends like Genny and Kris and Ron and God.

Don't be confused when I say God touches me and talks to me. My ears don't hear an audible sound. I don't physically feel a touch. Think how it is when one of your friends wants you to do something wrong; you know exactly what I'd tell you to do even if I'm not beside you. You've heard my advice in similar situations. You know me—what I'm like and what I want for you. That's the way I know God. He talks to me through the Bible verses I remember. What he said to people in the past is recorded in the Bible, and I know he'd say those same things to me if he were physically standing with me. I sense his presence in the same way you sense mine even when you can't see me. His presence is one strand of this story's pattern. The intermeshing of lives with God creates a special kind of beauty.

Just as the beauty of an afghan is enhanced by its practicality, so this book, written on one level to entertain, will be most valuable as it is useful to others. Everyone is touched by illness, their own, a relative's or a friend's. Faced with the crisis, we often panic, thinking, "I can't go through this." But of course we can and we do and we go on and forget the pain; we draw on the reserves that we've previously stored. Even though each person reacts uniquely, it helps to share others' experiences. This book provides vicarious experience for those directly and indirectly involved with cancer. It's meant to give information, comfort and insight.

Children take pride in showing off the needlework projects of their mothers. The value of the gift is greater when its beauty and warmth are shared and not hoarded away in a cedar chest. I am proud that you have chosen to share my gift to you with others. But never forget, Renae and Neil, that this is your book. No matter how many thousands of people share it, it will always belong to the two of you. Others will refer to the manuscript as *To Live Each Moment*, but our family will know that they're referring to *Renae's and Neil's Afghan*.

Love forever,
Mom

The Destroyer Returns

❦❦❦

FIGHTING THE ANESTHETIC, I STRUGGLED TO OPEN MY EYES AND clear my head. Genny hovered over me, waiting for my return to consciousness. "I guess I took advantage of my day to sleep," I sighed. "What time is it?"

"Two o'clock," came the answer from the other side of the bed —my husband, Rex. He was supposed to be hauling logs. We had both agreed that there was no reason to take a day off from the lumber company where he drove truck. I could ride with my friend Genny, who was going to Greenville Hospital herself for preadmission tests. She could have her blood tests and x rays while I had the small benign lump on my breast removed in outpatient surgery. Rex was supposed to be working.

Bewildered, I asked, "What are you doing here?"

"Genny called me. Dr. Coulter wants to talk to us both." He patted my shoulder. "How do you feel?"

"Sleepy."

"So what's new?" Rex gently ruffled my hair.

Smiling, I rolled my eyes. "You could hold the sarcasm at least until I get out of this place."

Twisting a blond curl onto his forehead was Rex's only sign of nervousness as he settled himself on the edge of my bed. "I'll get you home in a flash. The nurse went to tell the doctor you're awake." Shifting impatiently, he said, "I don't see why he couldn't have just talked to you and Genny without me."

Genny gracefully changed the subject. I lay viewing the familiar scene of my husband animatedly chatting with a friend. Searching his sparkling blue eyes, I wondered that, in spite of the twenty-five-minute drive to the hospital and the wait for me to wake, Rex had apparently not considered the reason he had been called.

But what Rex refused to see was instantly clear to me. Genny's sad eyes and my husband's unexpected presence clearly foreshadowed the purpose of our meeting with the doctor. His original diagnosis of a benign tumor had been wrong.

* * *

I had found the lump one late afternoon in March. Munching on a chocolate-chip cookie as I lay across our bed reading a novel, I dropped a crumb onto my neck. I sat up to brush it away, but it slipped into my bra. As I trapped the tenacious crumb, I paused. On the left edge of my breastbone was a barely perceptible lump —or was it simply an imperfection of the rib cage? I slid my hand to the right edge of the breastbone. I felt. No, the right side didn't seem to have that little hump. But the halves of our bodies are not perfectly symmetrical; my left foot is larger than my right. I wear a smaller ring on my left hand than on my right hand.

At that moment I wished I had followed the National Cancer Institute's advice on breast self-examination. I knew that early diagnosis and treatment are one's best chance for surviving cancer. Yet in spite of my knowledge, self-examination had remained one of those health habits that I never practiced—like exercising every day and avoiding junk foods.

And now, since I didn't know the normal shape of my body, I wasn't sure if I had a lump or not.

That evening as Rex and I undressed for bed, I mentioned the lump to him. "Would you check to see if there is a bump here on my breast?"

"Is this a new come-on?" He laughed, kissing the tip of my nose.

"No, smarty, I'm serious. I want to know if you think this is a lump or not."

"How am I supposed to know?" He withdrew, suddenly distant. "I'm no doctor. If you're worried, go see one."

"Really concerned, aren't you?" I snapped. "Remember, cancer is a good possibility with my family background."

"Now we're going to have a pity party, I suppose." Rex set his jaw and turned off the light.

I was angry and hurt. But after thirteen years of marriage and six years of dating Rex before that, I certainly should have known to expect his typical reactions to stress. Incidents flashed through my mind—Rex pretending to sleep in the chair in the labor room because he couldn't watch my discomfort—Rex hollering nervously at our son before stooping to cradle him and examine the depth of the gash on his forehead. I realized that Rex's curt dismissal of my possible lump was the same brusque masking of all his fears. But why, just this once, couldn't he have broken the pattern and alleviated my concern by discussing the lump?

"You're probably worried about nothing, as usual," he muttered as he turned away.

Attempting to view the situation objectively, I had to admit that Rex could be right. I was probably overreacting. Most of my friends had had lumps sometime in their lives, and, after the initial hysteria, all but one had found that the lump was simply a cyst or a benign tumor. I knew the statistics. Eight out of ten breast tumors are benign. I had little reason for alarm.

And I did tend to worry needlessly. For example, if Rex was several hours late from work and I'd had no word from him, I'd visualize him in a ditch under his overturned rig or in the middle of a five-vehicle pileup. Staring at the seemingly stationary hands of the clock, I'd agonize over rearing children as a single parent. I'd compute the possibility of keeping our farm with just my teaching salary, or I'd consider the advantages of moving to a small house in Greenville so that my mother could help with the children. Methodically, I prepared for widowhood until I heard Rex shifting down to back into our driveway with his tractor-trailer intact.

I reined in my wild imaginings as I remembered my tradition of panic. Rex was right. There was no reason to be afraid. But I would be prudent and get a doctor's opinion. I've always believed that the most paralyzing grief results from wondering, "What if I'd made her go to the doctor earlier? . . . What if I'd known that was a dangerous symptom? . . . What if . . ." I had vowed never to subject my family to the possibility of such guilt. The next morning, following the advice of my friend Genny who is a registered nurse, I dialed Dr. Frank Coulter, a general surgeon.

*   *   *

April 22, the day of my appointment, I dashed from the high school, where I teach English, to Dr. Coulter's packed waiting room. Initially every seat was occupied; several people stood shifting their weight impatiently. At last I found a chair and blocked out the noise around me to concentrate on grading papers. Eventually the nurse picked a chart from the counter and announced, "Janet Britton." As I followed her, I felt almost foolish for being there. Since the day of the cookie crumb, I had increasingly questioned my concern over such a tiny bump.

"Strip from the waist up," the nurse ordered as the examining room door slammed behind her. The sterile antiseptic smell intimidated me. My clammy fingers fumbled with the gown.

The doctor glided in. "Now let's look at the problem, Janet."

Dexterously examining me, he echoed my doubts. "I'm not even positive that is a lump. The breast is made up of glands and fatty tissue. You have very little breast tissue, so each gland is easily detectable."

"I never examined myself before, so I wasn't sure if that irregularity was normal or not," I apologized.

"Well, I'm sure there's nothing to worry about." His benign smile soothed me. "Make an appointment to see me in three months, though, just to verify that it is unaltered."

The flood of relief generated by his casual attitude shocked me. After the first evening's concern about the lump, I thought I had shoved the possibility of a malignancy out of my mind. On a conscious level, my only concern was protecting our seven-year-old and nine-year-old from the upheavals caused by our disturbed teen-age foster daughter. But nagging worry about the lump must have plagued my subconscious, for that evening I raced home and practically flew through my duties. Liltingly, I guided the children upstairs and tucked them in for the night. Later I floated into our own bed and nested against Rex. Brushing his head against mine, he asked, "Well, what did you find out today? Are you dying or anything?"

I ignored his teasing. "No, the doctor said not to worry about the lump; it's probably nothing. I have to go back in a few months, though, just to make sure. Looks like you'll have to put up with me a while longer."

"Always a smart remark," Rex chuckled, leaning over me for a good-night peck, and then snuggling peacefully against me as he drifted almost instantly to sleep. His relaxation paralleled my own sense of relief. The doctor's news was a reprieve. Our lives could go on as before—uncomplicated by illness. Waiting for my own sleep, I lay listening to my husband's rhythmic breathing.

* * *

Life was hectic in the months between my first and second examination. Our family survived the painful dissolution of the relationship with our emotionally ill foster daughter. Three weeks later Children's Services asked us to house Kris for the night, then for the weekend, and then indefinitely. Then summer arrived, and I began making the hour's trek to Youngstown State University to continue working toward my Master of Arts in English. Reading contemporary novels and writing papers for a literature course, digging in the library for obscure facts and memorizing thousands of trivial details for my research class absorbed my energy. The end of June slipped by. It was after my summer-school session in July before I thought to check my breast. The lump had not faded as had my conscious concern about it.

I called to set a day for a re-examination. No, it wasn't an emergency. Thursday, August 8, would be just perfect.

* * *

August 8 turned into my personal holiday. Kris volunteered to watch Renae and Neil for the day. Mom got a friend to watch her store, and we shopped, laughed and went out for lunch. I even treated myself to a hot fudge sundae—with whipped cream and nuts, of course.

Strangely, the waiting room was almost deserted when we arrived for my appointment. Before I had finished munching on my sundae, the nurse directed me to follow her to the examining room.

As I undressed, I thought, "What a silly interruption to a perfect day!"

Dr. Coulter strode in and had me stand on a footstool as he deftly examined me. "Yes, you were right," he said. "You do have a lump. It is much more distinct this time. Do you know what that means?"

I shook my head.

"It means that the lump has grown since April. I'm sure it is benign, but it's best to remove it now. I'll have the receptionist schedule you for outpatient surgery a week from tomorrow. After you wake up in the recovery room, you can go home."

I hesitated. He was moving too quickly.

"I hate to take the time to have the lump removed now. And if you're sure it's benign it seems needless to me."

"It'll just be half a day and a few stitches, and it is the most cautious approach. I'm so sure that it's benign that I'm not even going to plan for a possible mastectomy."

"Mastectomy?" I almost laughed. I certainly wouldn't agree to such radical surgery simply because he decided to schedule it.

As Mom and I left the office, I explained, "He's going to remove the lump next Friday—just to be safe." I couldn't read Mom's response.

A few minutes later, though, she casually said, "I was planning to leave Friday for Ken's wedding, but I think I'd better not go."

"Don't be silly," I argued. "You aren't missing your nephew's wedding. It's only minor surgery!"

*   *   *

The days before my outpatient surgery I scoured corners and hoed out closets. In only two-and-a-half weeks I would have to return to my teaching position. Graduate school and concern for friends had monopolized my time during the summer. Only a few days were left to catch up on the housework I'd neglected. The Thursday night before going to the hospital, tired from my spurt of domesticity, I decided that the last batch of peaches was still a little too green to process.

"I think I'll wait until tomorrow night or even Saturday morning to do these peaches," I commented to Rex. "Will you be home if I need help lifting the jars out of the pressure cooker? I may be a little sore."

"Of course, but your incision shouldn't bother you long. I don't plan to turn into a permanent maid."

"Don't worry. I never for a minute thought you were going to go domestic on me."

We both laughed at the thought.

The morning of Friday, August 16, I moaned and groaned and dragged myself to the bathtub. It was going to be a gorgeous day for a beach outing, and I was going to spend it in the hospital. What a bummer, as the kids would say.

Since I was having a general anesthetic, I had been instructed to ask a friend to drive me. I had followed the orders not to eat or drink anything after midnight, so by the time Genny pulled into our drive I was craving breakfast, even just a cup of tea. I closed the door quietly so as not to disturb Renae and Neil and Kris who were still snuggled in their beds. We stopped to get Helen, an older woman that the church calls Grandma, to give her an outing and to provide company for Genny while I was in the recovery room. Grandma Helen, who keeps three-fourths of the church's mending done and part of the community's as well, trotted down from her porch carrying her sewing basket.

* * *

I coasted glibly through the routine preoperative procedure. From outpatient registration I was directed to the lab and then to the x-ray department. I passed the time by discussing the educational requirements for each technician's job. I hoped that Kris could qualify for a program in the medical field as she had planned.

All too soon a nurse called me to be prepped for surgery. Sitting naked from the waist up in front of this stranger, I chattered about the first things that popped into my mind. I noted the irony of my having a lump removed just weeks after class discussions on the attitudes in the medical community toward women's illnesses. I babbled about the prevalence of prescribing tranquilizers and performing unnecessary surgery—especially hysterectomies. As the nurse dabbed my breast with Betadine, she noted the positive effects of an increase in women gynecologists and of the trend toward demanding second opinions.

I continued to rattle on. "I'm really fortunate that this lump is benign. The decision to have any form of mastectomy must be terrible. But then I guess reconstruction is becoming prevalent."

The nurse, working efficiently, pointed out that insurance companies still categorize reconstruction as cosmetic surgery. The reluctance of insurance companies to pay for reconstruction prevents many women from considering the operation.

The nurse and I were chatting like old friends by the time she left. I then passed time by scribbling a letter to Children's Services about arranging visits between Kris and her family. Mom popped in to say good-by before she left for the wedding. The nurse re-entered to medicate me for the simple surgery, and then she sent Genny in to keep me company until I was wheeled to the operating room. In the waiting room, Grandma Helen patiently patched the knee of a toddler's jeans.

* * *

I woke in recovery with Rex and Genny standing on either side of my bed. I knew then that Dr. Coulter had been wrong. The lump had been something to worry about. Thoughts cascaded in my mind. I won't react, I vowed. I will maintain eye contact and keep cool. I must get all the facts. I must support Rex. I must determine if Dr. Coulter is as honest as he seems. How will this affect the children?

"The lump was malignant. I want to admit you Sunday for a modified radical mastectomy." Dr. Coulter summarized the situation immediately upon entering the room.

"You said it was benign," Rex said, shaking his head in disbelief.

"I believed it was. It was small. And eighty per cent are benign. Janet just turned thirty-three and has had children. The evidence did not suggest a malignancy."

The room felt electrified. I pitied this surgeon who had to undergo our inquisition. But I began, "If it's in the early stage, isn't removing the lump enough? Isn't lumpectomy the current trend?"

"Lumpectomy is a new surgical procedure. So far its results are difficult to evaluate."

"Would the cancer research center in Buffalo, New York, suggest a mastectomy too?" I continued. "Would a second opinion agree on the need for the more radical surgery?"

"The mastectomy is the traditional technique," Dr. Coulter argued evenly. "It's proven. We've been using this procedure for years. We know that we can save lives with mastectomies. But we don't have statistics that conclusively show the effectiveness of lumpectomies."

A torrent of facts I had accumulated in reading and discussions rushed to my mind. "If there is no metastasis, the lumpectomy would be just as successful without the disfigurement."

The doctor remained firm in his position. "But we have no way of determining if the cancer has spread to the lymph system unless we remove the breast. We cannot analyze live tissue for metastasis."

I was frustrated to find that there were no conclusive answers to my questions—only varying professional opinions. My store of questions was depleted and I acquiesced. But Rex took up my defense. "Modern medicine, ha! Why do they have to mutilate to test if the cancer has spread? There must be a better way. It isn't right!"

Silence hung between the two men. Eyes locked in combat.

I felt like a medieval princess being attacked by a dragon while two knights argued whether to fight it with lances or swords. Both men were chivalrous. Both were searching for the best procedure to preserve my life. But I feared that they were about to forget the dragon and turn on each other. I feared that Rex, still outwardly calm, would explode to cover his fears.

"What happens after the mastectomy if you find the cancer hasn't spread?" Rex went on. "It's too late then to save her breast."

"Yes, you're right," Dr. Coulter admitted.

"In other words, thousands of women have gone through needless surgery."

Dr. Coulter charged ahead. "But surgery is the only way we have of knowing the extent of the cancer. Otherwise we're just guessing. And if we guess wrong, your wife will pay. We must know if there's node involvement to determine if further therapy is needed." And then he attacked with his strongest argument. "If there is no node involvement, physicians say a mastectomy results in over a 90% survival rate. That survival rate decreases to less than 50% if there is node involvement. And we must use all of the therapy available to assure women of that chance."

"There must be a better way," Rex repeated with a sigh.

"But there isn't."

Rex moved as if to shield me.

"This is a decision the two of you must make. I can only advise you and tell you, Rex, that if Janet were my wife, I would not risk the lumpectomy. We know that the mastectomy saves lives. We have perfected a very neat technique." The doctor hurled his final argument. "I would not risk a life for a breast. If you want to go for a second opinion, fine. Time is essential, though."

There seemed to be nothing more to say. Rex yielded. Dr. Coulter smiled reassuringly. "I'll schedule you for admittance

Sunday. If you have questions before then, call me at home. I'll be there all weekend."

"If she has no choice, admit her now," Rex pleaded with him. "Don't make her wait."

"I didn't allow for major surgery today. And I want to do several tests before the surgery."

I interrupted them. "I prefer having time to get used to the idea first anyway. It's much better this way."

Dr. Coulter smiled, almost gratefully. "Go get settled. Talk," he urged compassionately. "I'll see you Sunday."

*   *   *

On the ride home from the hospital, Rex suggested, "Relax a few minutes, honey. You'll need the energy to deal with the next few days."

I did close my eyes, but I couldn't sleep. Instead, just as I always did when I was upset, I conjured up my treasured storehouse of memories of my life on the farm. I sunk back, enveloped by a collage of childhood impressions.

Once more I hear the cows shifting as they graze in the pasture outside my bedroom window and the owl hooting down from the silo roof. Through the stillness of a summer's evening I hear the little frogs cry "knee deep," and one great bullfrog by the pond croaks like the man at church who always clears his throat during the organ prelude. I wake to the milk truck's scattering gravel and the John Deere tractor's putting. I pedal my bike leisurely to the cornfield where the morning breeze rustles through crisp stalks of corn, sounding like a parade of ladies in taffeta skirts, and I listen once again to see if Dad was right when he said that whenever the morning sun beams down after a refreshing rain, the corn complains of growing pains.

I summon back the weight of the blankets Mom piled us under on blustery winter nights. I recapture the memory of shoveling bag after bag full of seed oats while the dust stings our eyes, fills our noses and coats our mouths. I feel again the damp cool earth under my bare feet as my sister and I pad along the furrow behind the plow, picking up fishing worms. I thrash back and forth once more as the tractor pulls the lunging rake which scratches and pounds the ground while half-rolling and half-throwing the stalks of hay into windrows. As I drive down the field, the sun's rays beat upon my back, and as I return, they blister my face. And later, riding to the barn atop a wagon stacked six layers high with bales, I become a maharajah riding a huge, cumbersome elephant.

For the thousandth time I relish the aroma of homemade bread wafting up the stairs to my bedroom. Again I press my nose to the nose of a newborn puppy. The scent of roasting marshmallows and hot dogs mingles with the smoke of the bonfire of brush cleared from a new field. The fragrance of bouquets of wild-flowers from our woods—violets, cowslips, wild roses, daisies—floats through our sprawling farmhouse.

I remember the delicious raisins that I took from the cupboard in the barn to share with my pony, the tantalizing piece of candy (with the corner picked off to inspect the filling) that I chose from the five-pound box of Brach's assorted chocolates each Sunday from Thanksgiving to Christmas. And the scrumptious menus—warm milk freshly squeezed from the cow, mounds of fresh whipped cream on peaches or pineapple upside-down cake, and new potatoes and peas cooked moments after being picked from the garden.

Once again I wend down our dirt road, canopied by the trees' green boughs, to a small bridge where I pause to gaze at the lonely old carp drifting in the creek as the smaller bluegills dart past him. I re-envision the swaths of hay falling behind the mower like rows of giant green dominoes, stirring the scent that rises from the field. Once again our gnarled old plum tree excitedly waves her delicate white blossoms at me, and I mix dippers of tiny ladino, red clover, trefoil, timothy and alsike seeds into ever-changing kaleidoscopic patterns for Dad to bag and carry to the field to drill with the oats.

But then although the seasons do not change, nor the beauty, nor the family, a cloud of gnawing fear descends over this secure pastoral world. When my brother, sister and I reminisce, events are dated B.C. or A.C.—before or after Dad got cancer. This Friday afternoon, as I travel away from outpatient surgery, I want especially to shove aside the A.C. memories, but again they storm the defenses of my mind and rush in.

*   *   *

Dad had always been thin and prone to pneumonia. But when I was a high-school sophomore, my father's health progressively worsened. Mom force-fed him tons of "fat food"—giant sugar cookies, "sticky buns," biscuits and gravy, elderberry cobblers. She planned menus for a Goliath, but Dad continued to lose weight and strength. Because of the rigors of farm life, Mom urged him to return to an eight-hour-a-day job as a machinist, but months passed before Dad could bring himself to give up the land and the herd in which he had invested years of his life and go to work in a nearby shop. The cycles of planting and harvesting were broken.

Dad continued to weaken. His pants sagged on his emaciated frame, and a neighbor reported that Dad stopped each morning on his seven-mile trip to work to vomit along the side of the road.

Finally my father grew so weak that he had to be admitted to the hospital for observation. There it was discovered that Dad's temperature would climb to over 104 degrees and then break and start to rise again. The repetition of this cycle accounted for his repeated night sweats. But x rays showed nothing. The doctor asked Mom to give her permission for a team of surgeons to conduct exploratory surgery.

That evening I observed Dad as I would a stranger. Not until that moment did I see that the hard, callused, brown hands were bleached white with sweat. The rough, rugged hand that had brushed my cheek tenderly when Dad would pass me in the barn did not exist. No longer did he firmly grip me. Now his white hand—these skeletal fingers with foreign skin draped over bone —lay limply on mine.

I had convinced myself that Dad would soon be well and farming as always. Now I faced the facts—at six-foot-five-and-one-half inches tall, he weighed only 130 pounds. My father was dying.

I had avoided reshaping my mental picture of my father. I had always seen him as immortal as Mother Earth—an integral part of nature. If I were to paint a portrait to capture the essence of my father, I would picture him stooped in the dirt, still dressed in his Sunday suit, because every week after planting on his way home from church he would stop at the cornfield, take off his hat and amble to the second or third row. There he would kneel and gently prod in the earth until he found a faded and shriveled seed with a tiny white shoot sprouting from its tip. Dad—coaxing a calf from its warm womb, planting a tomato plant, fishing, gathering hickory nuts and walnuts. Dad—laughing at the county fair, Dad shadowed by his mongrel collie. Dad—his weathered, cracked hands awkwardly inching a blanket up over my shoulders in the middle of a January night. This father had been stolen away. In his place lay a ghostlike stranger.

$$* \quad * \quad *$$

Believing there was no other viable decision, Mom signed for the exploratory surgery. Outside the operating room hours dragged by as Mom and we children huddled, falsely cheerful for each other. While we waited impotently for news from surgery, the stark white walls glared ominously. The vinyl chairs squeaked as we repeatedly shifted our weight. My sister Bonnie and I giggled as a dyed-blonde fifty-year-old waddled to the elevator. Her garters, holding up nylons which fit like sausage casings, peeked out from under her skirt.

We were instantly sobered, however, by the appearance of the doctor, still dressed in his operating greens.

"We found the problem," the surgeon said. "A tumor as large as a grapefruit attached to the left kidney. We had to remove two ribs and part of another to get it all, but we did get it, and he should do just fine." He repeated himself. "We think we got it all."

Tears of relief streamed down my brother's face, my sister's face, and my face. Mom's face remained inscrutable as she murmured, "Thank the Lord. It's over. . . ." What our family did not know at that moment is that cancer is never really over.

We returned to our Before Cancer lifestyle, outwardly oblivious to the threat of a recurrence. The skeletal sweat-bleached hands again became brown and callused as Dad rebuilt a herd and cleared more woods for farmland. And the cycle of planting and harvesting began again.

But Dad's affinity for agriculture was not the only reason for returning to farming. As he explained in a letter to the unemployment office, he felt forced back:

> My former boss laid me off because the work he had for my machine was too heavy lifting. I have found that people do not seem too anxious to hire someone new who has had a recent serious operation when they think there is a possibility of recurrence such as there is in cancer. . . . As I was sick for 1 1/2 years before I had an exploratory operation and they found my trouble, it has affected my nerves and seems as now the pressures of life seem to bother me more than they should. I would like to just work and not be constantly reminded of my physical condition. It sort of puts a person's back to the wall.

Farming was Dad's way of escaping constant reminders of his illness.

*   *   *

I graduated from high school, enrolled in college and accepted a diamond from my high-school sweetheart, Rex, before he left for the Air Force. I directed my life toward the future. But if Dad got a simple virus, I would find myself haunted by the past's nebulous fears. I'd lie awake staring into the blackness, listening to the eight-track of questions that I could not escape.

What if Dad's illness is more than the flu? What if the doctors were wrong? What if they didn't remove all the tumor? What if Dad's return to health has only been temporary? Who will run the farm? How can Mom manage her store and take care of Dad?

What if Dad's illness is more than the flu? What about my own plans? How can I ever go through with our wedding plans if Dad is seriously ill? I can't possibly go overseas with Rex and leave the family. How can I choose between the man I am to marry and the man who has cared for me since I was an infant?

What if Dad's illness is more than the flu? How can I be separated from Rex indefinitely? How can I ask him to stay in Turkey alone, indefinitely? How can I risk our becoming strangers during months apart? And who can say how long Dad's illness will last? The uncertainty could stretch into years.

But it can't be more than the flu. I can't be asked to choose between my father and my fiancé. Certainly Dad is fine. It has been two years since Dad's surgery. He looks better than he has in years. Of course, he only has the flu.

But...

What if Dad's illness is more than the flu? What if the doctors were wrong? What if they didn't remove all the tumor? What if...

The tape continued to play. And the night passed. And another night passed. And soon the tape broke. Dad was fine once again. I returned home for another summer vacation.

* * *

In June, when daisies and vetch sprinkle the roadside and rabbits hop complacently down the narrow dirt road, Dad and I, after chores, drove to the field. A light dew had already evaporated. Dad mowed the center acres, the standing hay that remained, while I raked the outside swaths that had been mowed several days before. By the time we had finished a hasty lunch, the windrows would be dry enough to bale. "Summers are going to be more complicated for Dad with us children gone," I mused. "Mom and Dad are going to have to hire part-time help. That is, until their grandchildren are old enough to help." I chuckled to myself at the comment Dad would have made if he had heard my thoughts.

Dad interrupted my daydreams by motioning for me to stop the tractor and go to him. "Another breakdown," I moaned. "Too bad we can't afford all new equipment!"

But it wasn't the equipment.

"Do you see anything on my neck?" Dad asked. "Right here." He pointed to the base of the right side of his neck.

"Well, yeah, you do seem to have a bump there."

Unverbalized fear stood in the air between us. (It might be

cancer! But it mustn't be cancer. Certainly our family was over that paranoia by now.)

"A bump like that could be most anything," I babbled. "It doesn't look red. It's probably a welt from some insect in the hay. You know, sometimes you don't even feel them when they bite."

Dad's tanned face crinkled into a smile as he reached down and gave me a bear hug, stifling my flood of words. With my face crushed into his white T-shirt, I heard him say, "I've had a good life—no regrets. I just wanted a few more years with Shirley."

Dad agreed to go to the hospital for a battery of tests. My rugged, brown father didn't fit the sterile white hospital environment. The picture he made sitting in the chair that afternoon contrasted sharply with my image of him in a hospital bed two years earlier. His appearance now seemed to shout that he would be just fine.

The next day, after running last-minute errands for my wedding, I raced back to the hospital and discovered Mom slumped on a bench in the hall outside Dad's room. "What is it?" I asked, sitting down beside her.

Mom didn't answer immediately. I waited. "It's Albert." She paused and started again. "The doctor just said . . . he told me that . . . x rays showed a spot on your father's lungs. The lumps on his neck are swollen lymph nodes. The cancer has spread. But he's feeling good now and this is no time to tell him." I sat frozen as her words etched my brain. She pulled herself erect and marched into Dad's room.

I stumbled blindly in the opposite direction, bumping into a practical nurse who had graduated from high school with me. She steered me into an adjacent storage room.

"Dad has cancer," I choked. "There's nothing the doctors can do. And they're lying to him. And I have to act like nothing's wrong. And—" I sobbed.

"I know," my friend interrupted. "I just read his chart when I came on duty."

*   *   *

The next days drifted by in a haze. On automatic pilot, Mom

and I pretended all was well. Within days after his discharge, however, Dad's breathing became labored. Mom immediately wanted to call the doctor. Dad questioned her unusually quick response. "What's all the fuss over a bad cough?" he asked. "I just had a thorough checkup and I'm fine."

The cough lingered. Dad struggled to ignore it and his progressive weakness. He began to fret about his inability to keep up his former pace. Mom could not tolerate his feeling needless guilt. He had to know will power wasn't enough this time. Finally Mom told him. He was not shocked. He had been aware of the probability of cancer even though the doctor hadn't told him the facts.

Dad made it clear to Mom that he wanted me to go on with my plans. He didn't want my wedding ruined; he wanted me to be happy. He didn't want me to know how bad he was until I was married and in Turkey. Mom didn't tell him that I already knew.

In our conversations Dad tried to prepare me for learning about his cancer. His last words before Rex and I left for the airport were, "If you love me, love your husband and be a good wife."

* * *

I blocked the pain of that memory from my mind. I pushed away the thoughts of the After Cancer years. I fast-forwarded thirteen years to the car which was taking me from outpatient surgery to a household that would need shielding from the barbs of cancer.

I sighed and opened my eyes.

"Did you have a nice nap?" Rex asked.

I smiled.

* * *

The past faded, but the present bombarded me. So many people to prepare. So much to organize in just one day . . .

"How are you doing, Mom?" The children bounded out the door the second our car stopped.

"Fine. Just a little sore."

Renae and Neil ran off to play, satisfied, but Kris's eyes demanded more information. *I must tell her now. Then I'll rest,* I thought. Kris—how could we have brought her to our house to cause her more turmoil? We had dreamed of compensating for the previous instability of her life. And in the last few months, our love did seem to be salving her painful memories. Kris had begun to sleep without screaming awake from nightmares; she no longer jumped in terror when we woke her unexpectedly. She was being counseled by our minister and was attending church with us voluntarily. She was beginning to make new friends and had almost broken the ties with her destructive boyfriend. She had begun to develop trust in us—to risk saying that she cared about us. Would the nascent buds of trust be squashed? I was afraid that in the face of my illness, our idealistic dreams for her would evaporate like a vapor in July sun.

But we had accepted her as part of the family, not promised her paradise. It was time for her to learn that love is sharing—the good times and the bad.

I detained Kris with a glance. With the children safely out of hearing, I briefly explained, "I'm going back to the hospital Sunday for more surgery. The lump was malignant. But I'll be O.K. Don't worry. We'll get you graduated and settled."

Kris did not respond. I continued, "I'm afraid we'll be depending on you for a lot of help for a few weeks, though. Is that O.K.?"

Kris gave me a hug but said nothing. I should have known she would be outwardly calm. "I wish this weren't happening just when you're getting used to us," I said. "But then unfortunately you're probably more used to upheaval in your life than we are."

Kris fled to her room. She returned wearing a different blouse and combing her hair. Rex shouted to the little ones, "Hurry up or you'll be late for Vacation Bible School." They brushed my cheek with hurried kisses and ran to the car.

"Now I'll rest until tomorrow," I sighed, but as I passed the phone in the kitchen, I paused. Bonnie and Bud! My brother and sister who had suffered with me through Dad's illness must be told by me. I dialed Bonnie.

After the conventional questions of "How are the kids?" and "Did you can all your peaches?" I broached the immediate topic. "Bonnie, I have something to tell you, but I don't want you crying. Understand?"

"What a dumb thing to say. Of course I won't cry."

"My lump was malignant. I have to go in for surgery Sunday."

The telephone roared with silence.

"Bonnie, if you start crying, I'm going to hang up."

She sniffled. "O.K., O.K., just give me a minute."

Stroking her with my voice, I tried to soothe her sorrow.

The call to Bud was even shorter and more factual: I just wanted him to know what was going on. I'd be just fine. We weren't sure yet how to tell Mom. Yes, I loved him, too. I hung up, relieved that the ordeal of telling my sister and my brother was over. Other calls could wait.

I fell asleep almost the moment my body sprawled on the couch. When I awoke, the kids were in their pajamas watching television on the floor beside me. Rex smiled when he saw my open eyes. "Hi, sleepyhead." He ruffled my hair tenderly. "I'm glad you woke up in time to go to bed!"

We all went upstairs together. I moved cautiously, careful not to put pressure on my stitches. Rex settled the children and then came to bed. I cuddled against him and murmured, "Are you all right, honey?"

"Of course. I'm not the one who has to go through the surgery."

"You know what I mean!" A few minutes passed before I spoke again. "I don't think I'm surprised about the cancer. I always knew our family is high risk. But I really thought I'd be healthy at least until I was forty. With just the two children, I figured I'd be sure to have them raised if I did get sick. I didn't expect to be this young."

"No one is too young," Rex said. "Stanley wasn't too young." (Stanley, our neighbors' three-year-old, died of leukemia.) "Les wasn't too young." (Les, our dear friend, died of cancer at the age of twenty-nine, leaving a seven-month-old baby boy and a two-year-old daughter with his wife.) "Pam wasn't too young." (Rex's sister Pam, a cheerleader who had just bought her first pair of contacts and was making plans for a career as an airline stewardess, was killed in a freak car accident when she was sixteen.)

Rex was right. I certainly had no more claim to an extended life than these young people.

But as I lay beside my sleeping husband, staring out the window at the maple tree illuminated by our security light, I prayed, "Father, let me live in health just until the children are grown. Don't let them be scarred by my illness and death."

Surely God would understand my desire to rear my children. I wasn't begging to be healed for selfish reasons. I paused. "I love my little ones so much."

In the stillness I seemed to sense God touch my shoulder and whisper, "I love them so much that I gave my only Son so that they can live forever. And I gave them to you and Rex to train."

"I do appreciate your entrusting them to me, Father. But I'm having a hard time saying, 'Thy will be done.' "

He nodded empathetically. Tenderness and strength mingled, encouraging my trust. "Please teach me to be a good mother as long as I live. And no matter what happens to me, please continue to protect them."

*   *   *

I woke without an alarm.

One day, I thought. *I have one day to prepare a household for an indefinite illness. One day to prepare our children for rumors and fears.* The family must not be tormented as I was by my father's illness. I had to protect them from that.

By all outward appearances, it was just a typical summer Saturday at the Brittons. The children and I quickly cleaned the house. We canned peaches while Rex and a neighbor installed a door in our new entryway. Friends dropped in to chat. In the evening Kris went shopping, and the children and Rex and I munched on popcorn and watched television until bath time. As I watched the children skip up the stairs, concerns swallowed my thoughts: "What if I am not able to parent the children into adulthood? How will that affect them?"

I ruminated on the two cancer cases in my family—Dad and his mother. Dad died at forty-seven, four years after his illness began. But Dad lived every moment of those four years. When Grandma was in her early forties, she also contracted cancer. She recovered eventually and lived until she was seventy-three. Yet in a way she was dead for thirty years before the undertaker finally buried her. She was obsessed with bowel movements, with drafts which might result in coughs, and with "natural" foods. Driven by fear, she lost her productivity and her purpose for living.

In considering the effect of these two people on my life, I admitted that whether or not I died of cancer was not the most influential factor in my children's future; for if I lived to be eighty with an attitude like my grandmother's, I would destroy my little ones. But if I could instill a matter-of-fact acceptance of circumstances, then even my death would not critically wound the children's emotional lives.

Rex and I mulled over our approach to telling the children of my hospitalization. "You do the talking, Babe. You're better at explaining things than I am." Rex shrugged his shoulders. "Besides, I don't understand all the facts myself."

"No one does, unfortunately," I sighed. "I guess our own reactions are what's most important. If we're positive and honest, they'll do all right."

When I heard Neil closing his bedroom door after showering, I stood to go upstairs to tuck the children in. Rex took my hand, and we went together.

"Bring a Q-Tip so I can clean your ears," Rex called to Neil. "And Renae, finish brushing your teeth and come into Mom and Dad's room. We want to talk to you kids."

Sitting Indian-style at the head of the bed, I faced Rex. He wrapped his arms around the children, who sat on either side of him. "You heard that I have to go to the hospital tomorrow, kids," I said. "We want to explain everything tonight because Daddy will be with me at the hospital a lot."

"Oh, good," Neil laughed, "a family conference!"

"Listen carefully, Neil," Rex admonished. "We want you to ask any questions you have. It's important that you understand what's going on."

Neil bounced expectantly.

"You know what cells are, don't you, Renae?" I began.

"Oh, yeah, we had to draw them for science class. They have a nucleus and walls. That's all I can remember."

"Well, our bodies are made up of cells just like the plants and animals you studied."

The children's wide eyes revealed understanding.

"You know Mommy went with Aunt Genny to Dr. Coulter's yesterday to have that bump taken off. He had to make a little cut, and that's why I have this bandage." I showed the children the dressing on my breast.

"Does it hurt?" Renae wanted to know.

"Not really. It's just a little sore, but the doctor found out that the bump was made by bad cells. The bad cells kill the good cells so the doctor has to get rid of all the bad cells to protect the good ones." I began to get muddled. The children, though, didn't seem confused.

"I wouldn't want bad cells in me," Renae interrupted.

I laughed and forged bravely ahead. "The easiest way to get rid of the bad cells is to have surgery and take them away."

"You mean you'll have to have another operation?" asked Renae.

"Like on M*A*S*H!" Neil stated knowledgeably.

"Yes," Rex chuckled. "Only it'll be Dr. Coulter at Greenville Hospital instead of Hawkeye in Korea."

Neil looked puzzled. "Where do you have to have more surgery?"

"On my chest. The doctor thinks the cells might be in the rest of my breast, so he has to take more away or the bad cells will keep reproducing."

"Having babies," Renae explained to Neil.

"You didn't have to tell me," Neil grumbled. "I knew what Mom meant. What time are you going to the hospital?"

"After church tomorrow afternoon."

"Can we go see Grandma Durney?"

"No, she's at that wedding, remember? But we'll go out to lunch at McDonald's. How's that?"

"Yea! Can I have a large fries?" Apparently the educational lecture was completed.

"I guess so."

Renae asked, "Can I tell Dean to pray for you in junior church? We prayed for Cara's mommy when she went to the hospital."

"Of course, honey."

When the children were settled in their beds for the night, Rex and I snuggled together on the couch. "I notice you never used the word *cancer* when you were talking to the children," Rex said.

"That's true." I tried to summarize my views. "We must be honest with all the facts. But I don't want to use the catch-all word *cancer* until I have to. Some people are more shocked by that six-letter word than by any four-letter word. Their reactions would confuse and frighten the children."

"I don't know." Rex thought for a moment. "You might be right not saying *cancer* to the children, but it seems like you'll have to label your illness for adults."

"I just don't want to, honey. Remember how I hated dealing with everyone else's hang-ups when Dad had cancer? I want to try to save our family's energy to cope with our own emotions."

"But you can't keep secrets in a small community like this. I think you're wasting your energy trying."

"I won't try to hide that I'm having surgery. I just don't think I need to call a press conference to give medical bulletins to every casual acquaintance. We'll tell our friends the details—as we have the chance to see them."

"That won't be an easy job," Rex insisted.

"I know that. But when Dad got sick, people who never spoke to us suddenly sprouted from every corner to get the latest scoop —to be part of the drama of a terminal illness."

"Aren't you being a little cynical?"

"No, just realistic. I don't want the children subjected to that type of interrogation. And I don't want people peering curiously at my every move, circling like vultures surveying their prey . . ."

"O.K., cut the drama."

"Well, I might be exaggerating some. But I just want to live normally."

"You can't avoid the fact that our friends will be concerned about your health."

"People who love me are different. People who love me will accept me, well or ill, and treat me as they always have. They'll ask because they care about the answer, not to have something to add to the gossip."

"I guess you're right."

"Besides, I don't want the first kid I throw out of class to take bets on whether I'm missing my right breast or my left."

We both giggled.

*   *   *

I had not had insomnia since Dad's illness. But as Rex dozed fitfully at my side, my mind would not relax. Lists of people I should contact flipped through my head. I tormented myself wondering why Kris wasn't home yet. And an irrational guilt smothered me: How could I allow myself to get cancer? How could I subject my children, my husband, Kris to the emotional agony that cancer brings—the uncertainty, the terror?

An engine decelerated. I sat up and looked out the window by our bed. It was just our neighbor, returning late from playing his accordion in a Polish band.

I prayed for the peace of my family, for my mother's acceptance of my illness. I dozed.

I woke, glanced at the clock, and again ran through my fears. Is Kris in a hospital, in a bar, in a ditch . . . ? How will Renae and Neil be affected by my illness? . . .

I crawled out of bed. Perhaps the change in position would help me shake my thoughts.

"Where are you going?" Rex started, instantly awake.

"To the bathroom."

"Have you been sleeping?"

"Some."

"Get some rest for tomorrow."

"I'll try."

"I love you!"

I nestled back up to him and forced myself to lie still until he slept.

At 4:34 the car rolled up the driveway and slid to a halt on the gravel. *At least Kris is physically safe,* I thought. Banging doors, falling objects, general confusion—I forced myself to lie still and listen, fearing that if she had been drinking and I went downstairs before she was asleep, Kris would be either maudlin or argumentative.

When I had heard no sounds from downstairs for about ten minutes, I wiggled from Rex's embrace, gently shifting his hand from my shoulder to the bed without waking him. As I inched my weight from the bed, though, Rex roused and patted the hollow I had vacated. "What's the matter?" He bolted upright.

"Go back to sleep. Nothing's wrong. Kris is home. I'm just checking to see if the lights are off and the door's locked."

"Forget it. It's almost morning."

Ignoring him, I said, "I'll be right back." I had read too many stories about people who were drunk choking on their own vomit in their sleep. I had to assure myself that Kris was not lying on her back.

Like a small child, Kris, lying on her stomach, hugging her pillow and leaning against her stuffed bear, mumbled in her sleep. The world had been cruel to her.

"Father, please use these circumstances to strengthen Kris, our children, Rex, our friends. Don't let these days damage anyone!"

My mind, freed from the worries of immediate physical danger to Kris, began to relax. Drifting away, I talked peacefully with my heavenly Father.

Hospitalized

"I'M SO TIRED," I MOANED.

"Well, honey, don't worry about that." Rex grinned reassuringly. "You're going to have plenty of time to catch up on your sleep in the next month or so."

"Funny!" I heaved a pillow at him and darted to the hall to avoid retaliation.

Sunday morning—getting a family bustled off to church, playing the organ for the service—all was routine. But this day I was sensitive to every detail.

Sitting at the organ during the communion meditation, I observed our church family. So many times Rex had remarked that he was closer to the church family than to his biological family. An awareness that the same blood had been shed for each of our sins bound us closer than human bloodlines. Surely the love that holds the Church together is one of Christ's greatest gifts.

An impulse stirred in me to announce to all that I had cancer and needed them to watch over me and my family. I needed them to help bear my burden.

But then my eyes rested on the visitors and casual attenders. I couldn't face the gossip of acquaintances who wanted to be in on the latest suffering—leeches who lived vicariously on others' tears. I knew I had been right the previous night when I told Rex about my desire for privacy. I would not wear cancer like Hester wore her scarlet letter. Such added pressure I could not take.

*   *   *

Walking through the main door of Greenville Hospital a few hours later dredged up memories of the death of our stillborn child, emotions I thought had been blotted out by Neil's subsequent healthy birth. *I will not think about our baby's death,* I commanded myself. At that moment I wanted to think of the hospital as a haven of rehabilitation rather than a hall of death. Rex's eyes met mine and he smiled. Neither of us voiced the questions that hung between us. How long would it be before I could walk back out those doors? And would this be only the beginning of successive visits to the hospital, or would I be one of the fortunate ones?

To cover my apprehension, I joked with Rex. "I really don't understand why Dr. Coulter wouldn't go along with my suggestion and just burn my breast off like a wart."

Rex agreed, "It's obvious you're no Dolly Parton."

"I'm sure a mastectomy on me should be considered minor surgery," I insisted.

In reality, I knew all surgery had become much less serious. A ninety-three-year-old woman from our town had recently had cataract surgery and was discharged from the hospital the next day. Twenty years before, she would have had to lie flat with sandbags confining her for at least two weeks. And recently, just five days after her mastectomy, our neighbor had gone home with her staples (which sutured the incision instead of stitches) removed. I encouraged myself with this thought.

In the admissions office, outwardy I remained deliberately

nonchalant. Inwardly I fought a myriad of emotions. I casually answered the questions as the clerk typed.

"Reason for admittance?"

"Breast cancer."

"Which side?"

"Left."

The pert blonde typed without reaction. Such information was totally routine.

"My age? Thirty-three." My mind drifted. As a teen-ager I had believed that all significant life occurred by twenty-five. Now from a different perspective I thought, *I have so many things to do. I should have two-thirds of my adult life to live yet.* I mentally listed my goals. *I want to write a novel, to get my Ph.D., to spoil grandchildren. I want to finish remodeling our farmhouse, to take that trip to Great Britain, and to learn to swim. I want to influence young people in my classroom. And most of all, I want to train Renae and Neil until they are loving adults.*

"Lord, let me finish my work on this earth before I die," I prayed. "Lord—" My prayer was interrupted by the realization that thirty-three was Christ's age when he was crucified. How could I have the nerve to ask for more time to contribute to mankind than was given to Jesus, who had to meet the needs of an entire world? Did I deserve more time to work than the Son of God himself?

My reverie was broken by the secretary's next question. "What kind of perfume are you wearing? Is it Estee Lauder?"

I was amused at the abrupt change of topic. "You've got a fantastic nose!"

"Just for that one perfume," she demurred. "I love it."

"A friend gave it to me as a gift. A bottle seems to last forever."

As we returned to the lounge, I couldn't help thinking that it was so much nicer to discuss scents than to discuss cancer. If everyone were as accepting of my illness as this woman who works with disease every day, perhaps the open knowledge of my mastectomy would be as easy as Rex thought it would be.

An aide announced, "Janet Britton." Five of us stood. "Come with me," she said. "I'll take you to your room."

Unsure of her response, I declared my intentions. "I'm taking the children with me to show them where I'll be staying." I expected argument but got none—further proof that modern hospitals have changed policies.

As the children explored my room and helped me unpack, a nurse arrived to conduct a patient's interview. The questions amused me at first. When she got to asking how many bowel movements I had a week, though, I concluded that to survive a hospital visit one had to leave all modesty and dignity in the lobby.

When she left, at last, I sat twisting my plastic I.D. wristband and giving the children their final instructions. "You two take real good care of your daddy for me, O.K.? If you need anything, you may call, but try not to call more than once a day so we don't have a huge phone bill." We kissed and hugged, and Renae and Neil left, discussing their planned stop at the Dairy Queen.

"I love you," I shouted after them as I prayed, "Oh, let this be as simple as they believe it is."

I pulled Kris to me. "I know the kids drive you crazy sometimes, but I'm depending on you to take care of the family and the house." We clung together for several moments before she slipped from the room.

As the children disappeared I urged Rex to go with me to visit Genny, hospitalized one floor down. Friendship was a healing ointment to the worries blistering my mind. But my recess could not last. Sauntering back onto the third floor, I was immediately forced into my role as a patient. The nurse accosted me before I reached my room: "Would you please put your gown and robe on? We need to do some blood tests."

Ugh! The needles are starting, I thought.

While I was at the laboratory, Rex received word that my mother had returned from the wedding. He went to tell her of my scheduled mastectomy. Maintaining her usual outward composure, she handled this news as she had handled other sorrows of her life. No outward sign revealed the paralyzing fear that enveloped her at the sound of the word *cancer.* Her husband and now her child. The cycle repeating once again.

*   *   *

I was exhausted from the events of the last months—the full summer-school schedule, caring for troubled teen-agers as well as my own family, the shock of having our close friends Ann and Ron separate after nineteen years of marriage, and the further tension created by Ron's decision to sell the cattle and move to Virginia to attempt a reconciliation with his family. My fatigue was compounded by lying awake listening for Kris to stumble home from a binge that had undoubtedly been precipitated by my illness. But this first night in the hospital, in spite of my tiredness, once again I could not fall asleep. I phoned my grandmother and talked as long as I decently could. I called home and Kris told me that the little ones were in bed and Rex had gone to talk to the neighbor whose wife had recently had a mastectomy. I hoped the visit would encourage Rex. But even if it didn't, I was reassured that Rex wasn't bottling up his feelings.

Next I decided to read. I pulled Faulkner's *As I Lay Dying* from my suitcase. The title unnerved me. I put it down and chose a biography of Einstein. The squish of nurses' shoes and the rustle of starched uniforms signaled the shift change. I couldn't concentrate on my book. I tried to read the Bible. The words swam before my eyes. I talked to my Lord. "I know you can give me strength to face anything. But I just feel this is all impossible right now." A nurse walked in for her first rounds of the evening. Quickly, I wiped my eyes.

"Do you want to talk?" She issued the pat question in the appropriately concerned tone of voice.

"No, not now. Thank you." I, too, answered appropriately, but I thought, "Not until I'm sure yours is more than textbook concern to be recorded on my chart." I would save my true feelings for my family and friends.

Old memories revived. When Dad got cancer and my friends were playing the top ten hits of the week, I formulated my own top ten list—the top ten methods of dying. I carefully thought out my chart:

1. Taken, like Elijah, in a chariot of fire.

2. Cerebral hemorrhage.
3. Massive heart attack (while sleeping).
4. Hit and killed instantly by impact from a Mack truck (which I didn't see coming).
5. The bursting of an unsuspected aneurism.
6. The movement of a blood clot to the heart.
7. Carbon-monoxide poisoning.
8. Unexpected bullet wound to the back of the head.
9. Bitten by an asp (without realizing it).
10. Standing in the exact target of the first nuclear bomb of a surprise attack.

I had no doubt that cancer would never appear in any position on my top ten chart. In fact, if I ever took time to compose my ten least favorite methods of dying, cancer would top that list. (Well, after deliberation I might move it to second place and give the number one position to "Being burned alive.") To be dead was not frightening to me. The process of death was what I wished I could avoid, so every form of death on my top ten list was immediate.

I analyzed the term *cancer victim*. It elicited the image of an innocent bystander being smashed by a giant semi labeled CANCER, INC. Like an innocent bunny staring helplessly at the blinding headlights, the cancer victim stands frozen waiting to become a blood-and-fur blob on life's freeway. But I knew this image was false. Death by cancer is not the violent, instantaneous death of the rabbit. Death by cancer is lingering, unspectacular. It is like the death of a fly groping pathetically on a windowsill after its wings have been plucked by a bored eight-year-old.

I believed I had the courage to steel myself for a moment's agony in a violent demise. But the idea of contending with a lengthy debilitation that prevented my living life fully horrified me. I dreaded the thought of vivisection—painfully existing while my body is hacked, a piece at a time, and filled with poisonous chemicals. Living with cancer is like enduring the Chinese water torture—the steady dripping away of strength. Waiting for the next drop would drive me mad.

I sighed, deliberately pushing my mind's brake. In the momentary silence, I became aware of One insistently calling, "Child!"

"Yes, Father?"

"Peace I give to you; not as the world gives, do I give to you."

I tried to listen to him. But instead a nagging sense of futility returned. "I'm so tired. I can't fight this battle."

But he gently insisted. "Lo, I am with you always, even unto the end of the world."

I guess that includes a hospital bed, I admitted.

He prodded me. "Remember, child, whatsoever things are lovely . . . think on these things."

* * *

"Mrs. Britton, you're scheduled for a bone scan this morning."

Rubbing the sleep from my eyes, I staggered into the bathroom. As I dragged myself back to bed, the nurse returned with a specimen jar in her hand.

"That jar better not mean what I think it does," I moaned.

"We need a urine specimen before you have your bone scan."

"You're just about two minutes too late."

"Well, let's go downstairs. With the extra time maybe you can get a specimen for me."

I had no idea what to expect from a bone scan. The name sounded sinister. The purpose, to detect if the cancer had spread to the bones, seemed foreboding. But I knew nothing of the procedure.

"I'm an avowed coward. Is this painful?"

"No, there's nothing to it," the nurse declared in a chipper voice.

Her answer didn't relieve me, though, since a full three hours before I gave birth to Renae, nurses assured me that labor would be "just a little longer." And as nurses prepare to ram a foot-long needle practically through an arm, they traditionally warn, "Just a little pinch now." Well, I hoped this nurse's answer was factual and not sugar-coated.

Downstairs, I was handed a glass of water and the specimen jar. "There is one patient ahead of you. Just take your time." (Yeah, as long as my time comes within the next ten minutes, I thought.)

I was directed to sit in a straight-backed chair in a dressing cubicle. I stared at a door labeled *Hot Laboratory: Caution Radio-active Materials.* Soon I concluded that the only hot thing in there was the coffee the technician guzzled as she ate her doughnut.

As she chewed, my mouth watered and my stomach growled. I forced my eyes away from food to peruse the wall. Certificates in nuclear medicine technology, radiologic technology and clinical pathology leered back at me.

Five glasses of water and one half-hour later, I still could not urinate. The technician, on her second cup of coffee and third doughnut (could I be sentenced for contributing to the delinquency of a glutton?), asked if I had "had any luck."

"I think I've got a mental block about this whole thing."

"We only need a few drops. But I must have it before I can give you the injection."

Trying to make conversation, I asked, "What do you do? Check the level of a chemical in the urine before and after the injection?"

"No, we have to ascertain that you are positively not pregnant before we inject the dye."

I began to giggle hysterically. "Would the fact that I had a tubal ligation several years ago affect the need for this test?"

"You what? Why didn't you tell the nurse upstairs?"

"The surgery is on my records, and I had no idea why you needed a urine sample."

I wondered if this confusion was typical of medical bureaucracy. (I found out, in the next few weeks, that it was.)

Wearing white plastic gloves, the technician handed me two pills in a paper cup. The thought crossed my mind, "What does she think will happen to her if she touches these things?"

Increasingly, I was determined to know the reason for each step of the procedure. "What are these pills for?"

"To block the thyroid so it won't absorb the radiation."

Mmm, I wonder how the rest of my body views remaining defenseless while the thyroid gets special protection.

Fifteen minutes passed. The technician returned, sat down and recited her speech: "We are going to take pictures of your bones.

In order to do that we are going to inject you with a small amount of radioactive material. It will just involve a pinch—like a blood test. You will return in three hours. The test itself will take about an hour and a half. The only requirement from you is that during the next three hours you need to drink five to eight glasses of water. It may be in the form of tea, coffee, orange juice or any other liquid. Do you have any questions?"

The technician tightened the tourniquet on my arm and began injecting the dye before the bombardment of information had time to reach my brain. I became slightly nauseated, but I couldn't decide if it was a physical or a psychological reaction.

Three hours later I sloshed back downstairs. A second technician greeted me with the question, "Would you like to step into the bathroom first?" I grinned to myself. Either my water level was showing in my eyeballs or this was a usual problem.

The technician directed me to stand in front of a large round machine. She raised it up and positioned my chest against it. I watched as she stepped to a control panel and set a timer. "You may breathe but try not to move," she said as she pushed a final button. When the buzzer sounded about a minute later, she repositioned me. We repeated this procedure about fifteen times until she had taken a complete set of pictures of my bones from my skull to my feet.

While the technician worked, she noted, "You must have been conscientious about drinking plenty of water. Water clears the soft tissue of the radioactive material and improves the quality of the scan. And these are excellent pictures."

"I'd like to think my svelte figure permits a better view of my bones. But probably the actual reason is that I had a good head start on the water this morning." And I explained to her about the morning's incident.

That afternoon when I was sent for a mammogram there was another foul-up. I dreaded the mammogram as I always dread the unknown. My apprehension was increased by my deep sense of modesty. As soon as I entered the examining room, the technician locked both doors. (Was it to protect my privacy or prevent my escape?) While she readied the equipment she chatted, and I began to relax.

Then she described the procedure: "I'll ask you some questions and then I'll take four pictures—two while you're sitting on this stool and two while you're lying on the examining table."

She filled out a routine medical history: Is there any history of breast cancer in your family? Do you have children? Did you nurse your children?

I wiggled nervously on the stool. She adjusted the height of a stand to the base of my breast. Then I bravely slipped the gown from my shoulders. She turned and stared at me quizzically. "What is that dressing for?"

"I had surgery to remove a lump last Friday."

"Then there are sutures in that breast?"

"Yes."

"I sure hate to do a mammogram on that side. With your recent incision, it'd be painful to put pressure on that breast."

"Why would you need to take pictures of that side?" I was confused. "It won't be there tomorrow and the doctor already knows there's a malignancy."

"But he has scheduled a bilateral mammogram."

"I'd be glad to take the responsibility for refusing to let you do the left side." Silently, I determined that I would not subject myself to unnecessary pain. I would defend myself and not, lamblike, follow foolish orders.

Sensing my inflexibility, the technician reached for the phone. The doctor quickly verified that the order was an error. He had ordered a mammogram and the nurse had automatically written "bilateral," since that is the usual procedure. Again I learned that a patient must defend herself; not to question might result in a careless mistake.

My anxiety about the mammogram had been needless. The process was painless and quite simple. The technician rested my breast on the stand and directed the machine over it. The most uncomfortable part was twisting my head back out of the machine's view. A clear plastic device was used to flatten my breast. Since the pressure was even, there was no great discomfort. Next I was laid on my side on a cold examining table. Again compression was applied. After positioning me for each picture, the technician hid behind a shield and ordered, "Take a breath and hold it. . . . Breathe now."

*   *   *

I was shuttled about all day for testing. Rex raced in immediately after work, and we both settled back to relax. We had to interrupt our rendezvous, though, to sign releases. Yes, we understood the extent of the surgery. Yes, we understood that a skin graft would be necessary since there is not enough excess skin to cover the incision. (What a nice way of saying, "because you're as skinny as a rail.") No, we had no more questions about lumpectomies. The test results will be back Thursday? Fine. We're glad you don't expect any metastasis. Yes, we were fortunate that we found the lump in an early stage.

And then I was alone. Sleep! I needed to rest to fight back against the marauding cells. I wanted to be back home baking sugar cookies for my children instead of having nurses wait on me.

Within minutes after dozing off, I started, abruptly alert. "What time I am afraid, I will trust in God." Afraid—I had avoided that word. I had done a pretty professional job of maintaining my cool. But I now had to admit that my outward calm was all show, and God wasn't fooled by my coping role.

"Man looks at the outward appearance, but the Lord looks at the heart."

O.K., it's true. I'm terrified of repeating Dad's illness. I hate the idea of being an invalid.

"Fear not. My strength is made perfect in weakness."

Well, it looks as if you're going to have the perfect opportunity to show your strength.

God grinned at my attempted joke. He cradled me. I nestled closer to him.

*   *   *

I jerked awake. A nurse stooped over my bed. "I need to begin prepping you for surgery. Which side do you want your injection on?"

I dozed until a second nurse instructed me to step into the shower to scrub down with a sterile solution.

"You mean my left side?"

"Yes."

"But that doesn't make any sense, to scrub my sutured area."

The nurse hesitated and then agreed. "Just forget that for now. If they want, they can prep you for surgery after you're under." She shaved my left thigh, the donor site for the skin graft, and spread Betadine solution over it.

"I'll be glad to get this over with," I sighed. "I want to get home to paint the woodwork."

The hypo did not seem to make me drowsy. I fought its effects, wanting to remember every detail. Attended by my family like a queen being escorted to a royal audience, I was physically lying on a hard cart. But emotionally I was cushioned by love.

Parked for an interminable period in an anteroom, at last I was wheeled into a cold vault. The ceremonially gowned automatons of the operating room appeared oblivious of my presence. The drone of their conversation was interrupted by one mechanical voice directing me, "Slide onto the table, please." Naked under my thin cotton gown, I felt like a participant in an ancient rite of human sacrifice, the victim forced onto the sacrificial stone by these priests of the operating room. Metal instruments positioned on a gleaming tray substituted for the traditional flint knife. I submitted stoically as my breast was bared (to cut the heart from the live victim). The anesthesiologist pulled my right hand to the right side, and my left arm also was extended and strapped so that I would not reach out to impede the downward thrust of the knife. The blood offering awaited only the arrival of the high priest, the surgeon.

Again backs were turned toward me.

Dr. Coulter entered, all dressed in green like the medieval knight who fought Gawain. And I remembered that although the Green Knight spared Gawain's life, yet his axe permanently scarred Gawain's neck. My Green Knight's attempt to save my life would also leave a scar that would always remind me of this encounter.

"I'm going to put you to sleep now. Count backwards from 100."

* * *

Voices filtered into the mists of my consciousness. My leaden eyelids parted a slit. I saw the gleam from metallic carts skating over the crystal tile in a frosted-white room. I strained to ask what time it was, but my swollen tongue would not articulate. One back revolved. "You're in the recovery room," shouted a nurse who seemed suspended in another dimension. Her voice echoed in this frozen tundra. I tried to smile to convince her I was alert, but my dry lips would not curve. I succeeded only in baring my teeth in a distorted grimace.

"Janet, take deep breaths."

Yes, I must. Pain stifled my attempt. But I must.

I cracked my eyes quizzically as I felt my blanket being lifted and heard the placating voice, "You're doing fine. I'm just checking your dressings."

"I'm cold!" I fought to clean the film from my brain. It was like wiping steam from the bathroom mirror. I could see clearly for a moment and then slowly the haze crept from the corners and fogged my vision.

Once more I wiped the steam and became aware of the rocking motion as I was wheeled back to my room. I was a child again, swaying on top of a wagon piled six high with bales. Oh, to be warm like that again! My sweaty body was covered with biting hay and chaff. My shorts were handprinted with grease. My hair was tucked under a floppy straw hat.

No—no warmth. Instead I lay in a snowdrift, in my shorts, making snow angels. The damp cold permeated to the bone. No mirage of summer could erase the pervasive chill.

I stirred again. Backs had been replaced with eyes. Rex ran his finger over my shoulder. Mother caressed me with her eyes. My heart was warmed by the glow from a halo of love, even though my body was still icy.

I wanted to convince my family that I was fine—not to worry. But I could not sort the words I needed. I sighed resignedly,

"I'm so drowsy!"

Rex brushed the hair from my clammy forehead. "Just rest, honey. You don't need to talk. We'll be here when you wake up."

* * *

Years ago, it seemed, I could lie in bed and sleep as contentedly as Carnation's cows. Now each moment was torture. Certainly there must be a comfortable position, I thought. Each nurse who came into my room devised her own method of propping my pillows or adjusting my arm. But nothing seemed to relieve the agony.

My arm, shoulder and chest were not the only areas of pain. The donor site on my left thigh burned, as sensitive as if the ends of all the nerves were exposed (as they probably were). My bladder continued to swell like a balloon as the intravenous fluid infused. Surely the pain in my back and legs would lessen if I could just go to the bathroom, I thought. For a while I napped.

I woke again in pain from the breast incision and the bladder pressure. I attempted to move my leaden left arm, wishing I could free my right arm from the I.V. unit. "I have to go to the bathroom," I told Rex. The nurse answered my buzzer and removed a bedpan from the stand by my bed. Lifting my body onto the bedpan shot pains through my left side—my chest and arm and the donor site on my leg. But I couldn't shake the fear of wetting the bed. The attempt was futile.

"Using a bedpan should be part of pre-op training," I joked.

As the I.V. flowed, my discomfort increased. The pain in my back sliced down my legs. My full bladder seemed the only possible cause for my back cramps.

"Please may I get up and walk to the bathroom? I know I could go if I just had my feet on the floor!" I insisted.

After removing the plastic I.V. bag from its perch, two nurses steered me the nine long steps to the toilet. I fought to retain consciousness. Deep breaths and running water helped me dribble, but I had no relief. Discouraged, I was maneuvered back to my bed, readjusted, reconnected. I panted. My beating heart vibrated my dressings.

Time passed and my discomfort escalated further. The bedpan remained unused. The journey to the commode became increasingly treacherous. The room swirled around me. By midnight, a great whirlpool threatened to suck me under. A nurse arrived. "We must catherize you," she said.

I hesitated. "Can't you wait? I'm sure I'll eventually go by myself."

Gently ignoring my request, the nurse injected a hypo. "You'll feel much better with a catheter in place."

I acquiesced, humiliated at my inability to direct my body. The end of the water balloon was opened. The stomach and back pressure became less acute. I covered my embarrassment with a feeble joke. "You're just adding another tube to my collection," I said.

But some cramping remained. The nurse returned with a small package. Like a child having its diaper changed, I submitted to the nurses' adjusting a feminine napkin between my legs. What a mockery—this reminder of my womanhood on the day my femininity was permanently scarred.

The nurse left my room. Repeatedly I tried to pray. I needed to talk to God, my closest friend, as I normally did. I needed to share my reactions and doubts with him and listen to his comfort. But after a few sentences, my mind drifted. I pulled my straying thoughts together. "Father, I know I should pray specifically, but I'm too tired to talk now. Please just hold me until I feel better. Pat me."

"I love you, my child!"

"Abba!" Overwhelmed by helplessness, I now understood that name for God. I wanted to curl up on the lap of my Father in heaven.

* * *

On the left side of my bed, the sign clearly warned, "No Vein Punctures or Blood Pressure on Left Side."

The night shift came on duty. A nurse checked my dressings and the drainage in the hemovac, the plastic collapsible canister, about nine inches in diameter, which was attached by tubing to the incision extending from my chest wall through my armpit. Then she reached for my left arm to take my blood pressure. "No," I stopped her. "There's a sign on the wall." "I'm sorry. I didn't see it," was her flustered response. I dozed fitfully, trying to block the pain. Momentarily I nodded off. My eyes flew open. A lab technician stood on my left side, ready to puncture me for a blood sample. "You can't take blood from that arm!" I shrank from her, sending pain through my arm and chest. "The I.V. is on your right side," she coolly explained while continuing her preparations. "I had a mastectomy," I insisted. "There's a sign on the wall." She directed her flashlight on the sign and then hurriedly gathered her equipment to move to the other side. "Oh, I didn't notice it in the dark." She fumbled apologies as she contemplated how to penetrate the web of tubes on my right.

∗   ∗   ∗

I awoke for the hundredth time since the midnight shift began. Light streamed through the window by my bed. My roommate greeted me. "You won't be getting up by yourself to wash up, will you?" she asked as she eased into her robe. "No, not this morning." (*I wish I were.*) Overwhelmed by a sense of helplessness, I watched her glide to the bathroom. I listened to the water running. Brushing teeth, washing a face, eating a meal seemed absolutely impossible feats of courage. An age ago I stumbled through this morning routine like a sleepwalker. Now I was a prisoner, shackled to my body's weakness. My roommate sailed back to her bedstand for her shampoo. I asked her to phone my mother and ask her to stop on her way to work.

I lay passively amidst the bustle of morning hospital routine— temperature, blood pressure, pulse rate. The aide reached for my basin and toothbrush. I was embarrassed by my dependency. She sponged my hands and face and held a cup so I could rinse my mouth. The breakfast trays arrived. "I'll be back to help you eat when I'm done passing out the trays," the young aide cheerfully volunteered.

I was grateful for her casual warmth. "Thanks, but my mother will be here in a few minutes."

Mom lived only four blocks away. Eons had passed since my roommate had called her. My roommate finished her breakfast. A starched erect practical nurse removed her tray and frowned at me with disdainful reproof. She peered dramatically under the cover on my tray and chided, "Don't you know we have to eat to get better? Will we want our tray removed without our having a single bite?" I was taken aback. I hadn't realized that the stereotyped "we" medical staff still exist. I hoped the species would soon be endangered.

The cheerful aide bounced through the door and the starched tyrant began rhetorically, as one talks to a pet or to a car that won't start. "This young lady won't eat her breakfast. Now what should we do about that?"

I stopped her act. "You don't need to do anything. My mother will be here in a minute to help feed me."

"That's just what we need around here—an overprotective mother," she snapped.

I was weak but still had some adrenalin on reserve. No one attacks my mother in my presence. I mustered the energy for one sarcastic retort. "Aren't you compassionate? A real Florence Nightingale!"

The starched one retreated without comment.

I continued to fume even though she was gone. How did she expect me to tolerate the pain and maintain enough coordination to feed myself a whole meal with my left hand? My right hand was attached to a board and connected to the I.V. unit. If I did manage to grab a fork, I'd be terrifed of hearing the I.V. buzzer signal that I had disrupted the needle and blocked the flow of the fluid. I did not want to disturb this site. My goal was to have Dr. Coulter remove the I.V. bottle before the needle had to be relocated.

I could not demean myself to ask for help from this stranger. I hated being a case—a chart and not an individual. With her bully's personality, no wonder she chose nursing, I thought. It's easy to intimidate a person on a bedpan or one whose survival depends on tubes and bags. Pressed and starched and perfumed, of course she can feel superior to sweaty, disheveled patients who lie with thin hospital gowns tied to necks and tangled under armpits.

The click of heels down the hall signaled my rescue. The calvary arrived in a regiment of one—my mother. Quietly, unassumingly she kissed my cheek and smiled. Then without comment she marched to the nurses' desk to trade the coffee for tea. Knowing my preferences and reading my body language, she fed me as she once had when I was a little girl. I felt the same security. As if I were curled on my mommy's lap, I told her how the nurse had made me feel like an object. "I don't need someone to humiliate me in order to get me to fight back to health. Dad forced himself to eat and so will I. I'm going to build up my strength and go home to my family."

Mom listened to me without interrupting. Then she dropped a few seeds of wisdom. "I'm sure the nurse did what she thought was good for you. Don't waste your energy being upset with her."

After I finished gagging down my toast, I lay back, exhausted from the effort. Mom expertly freshened my face with warm soapy water, fluffed the pillows under my head and readjusted the one under my arm. She changed the angle of my bed and wrapped a flannel blanket around my clammy feet. How many thousands of times had she attended to my father so gently? I wondered. To me, soothed by her love as well as by her physical care, she exemplified the virtuous woman of Proverbs: "Her children arise up, and call her blessed."

"I'm so blessed to have you here, Mama!"

*   *   *

My goals were simple—eating and moving by myself. If I could gain independence, I could go home.

Another practical nurse, Sarah, and an aide arrived to change my bed and take me for a walk. Efficiently they helped me sit on the edge of the bed and dangle my feet for several minutes. While they clipped the catheter bag and hemovac, I fought the black clouds that were blowing across my mind.

"You must feel as if you're working in geriatrics," I said. "This is quite some feat."

Euphoria swept over me as I stood and took my first step. I was confident. I would walk the halls and the doctor would remove the tubes. I would soon be strong again.

"This is going well," I gloated to Sarah.

* * *

I was slumped over the edge of a chair. Ammonia burned my nostrils.

"Why didn't you warn me you were going to faint?" Sarah nervously chided.

"Is that what I did? I wasn't planning to."

"You took us by surprise," the aide stammered. "We didn't know where to grab you."

* * *

That afternoon the strong farmgirl-turned-nurse returned with her reinforcement. "You need a walk before we go off duty," Sarah encouraged. "This time we're prepared." The robust one laughed as she held out three ampoules of smelling salts. Again the hemovac and catheter were clipped and the I.V. unit was positioned to be pushed ahead of us. I was dangled over the edge of the bed in preparation for launching.

Sarah issued my last-minute orders. "Remember. Don't look down. Don't close your eyes at all. This time we're going to make it!"

Staring into Sarah's determined eyes, I stood and took three steps. I fought to retain consciousness. Blackness crept over my vision. My ears roared. I took another step.

* * *

I woke sitting in the chair. My eyes watered from the acrid ammonia scent. I grinned weakly and closed my eyes to rest for several minutes.

I had become a challenge to Sarah. "Before we put you in bed, let's try again," she suggested.

I propped my eyes open and stared ahead. I fought the clouds, the mists that threatened my consciousness. I strained to see as my vision blurred. I struggled to hear over the roar in my ears. Sarah waved smelling salts under my nose with each step.

"Just a few more steps before you turn," she encouraged. "You're doing fine. . . . Keep going."

My toe touched the hall tile. I wobbled. Slowly, she swiveled me back toward my bed. "We made it!" she exulted.

I was arranged in bed and medicated. I closed my eyes to rest.

"Now I can write on Janet's chart that she was walking in the hall," Sarah told the aide as they left.

I smiled. We all have our own personal goals, I thought.

* * *

Thursday, two days after my surgery, Rex brought the children to visit me. We agreed it was important for them to see for themselves that I was O.K., so that their imaginations wouldn't have free rein. Mom brushed my hair and helped me apply a touch of blush and lipstick. I discreetly covered the hemovac with the sheet and had the bed cranked to a comfortable sitting position.

Rex had prepared the children for the I.V. and tubes. They tiptoed into the room. "How do you feel? When will you be home?" were the first questions out of their mouths.

I warmed at the arrival of these ambassadors from my normal life. Looking at them, I could believe that life would go on unchanged. As the children relaxed, they gained animation, telling me stories of the four days that had passed since I entered the hospital.

Kris sat on a chair, inscrutable. When the children ran down the hall for a drink at the fountain, I summoned energy to draw her out. "How are you, honey? How are things going at home?"

"I'm all right. Everything's O.K." Her eyes remained veiled. She talked of events but not of her emotions. I could not crack her stone mask.

"I don't know what we'd do without you."

Her face softened. For a moment I imagined she would tell me what she was really thinking.

The little ones scampered in. Neil plopped on the bed to hug me. He landed directly on that plastic container called the hemovac. Startled, I jerked back. His eyes popped open in fear. I tried to calm us both. "You didn't hurt me. This little thing collects the fluid from where they did my surgery. You just surprised me."

Renae and Neil hesitated to touch me after that. Their lips barely brushed mine in a kiss good-by when Mom came to take the three of them back home.

After they were gone, Rex shook his head. "You shouldn't have tried to hide that thing. I think those kids are pretty tough. The drainage probably wouldn't have bothered them as much as it does you." With all my speeches about straightforwardness, I had frightened my little ones by trying to hide reality.

The visit had exhausted me. I napped as Rex, with his hand resting on my shoulder, watched television and talked to my roommate. The pressure of his hand comforted me.

* * *

I woke to the sound of Dr. Coulter's and Rex's laughter. Seeing my eyes open, Dr. Coulter said to Rex, "I hear your wife has been keeping the nurses alert on their walks."

I joined in. "I just love all the attention," I confessed. "I feel important when I wake up surrounded by the floor's entire nursing staff."

He grinned, examined me and bustled on to the next room. After he had left, I thought, *He never said anything about the lab report. I'm sure he said he would have it by today. I wonder if he is avoiding the topic or if the report is late.* But I didn't mention my doubts to Rex. It was no time to dwell on possibly imaginary problems.

* * *

Later that night I woke to the light of a flashlight as a nurse padded into my room to check my dressings.

"I feel so much better tonight," I told her. "I've slept almost normally."

Discussing the weather and her daughter's upcoming wedding, the nurse adjusted the pillow under my left arm, smoothed my blankets and poured fresh water. She moved gently and efficiently, anticipating my needs just as my mother did.

"You are so sensitive to the little things that make me more comfortable. Thank you."

The nurse lowered her eyes shyly.

I continued, "I have a theory that a good nurse has either been sick herself or has taken care of someone close to her that was seriously ill. I think maybe it takes personal experience to understand the frustrations of illness. You never make me feel infantile. I never have to prove anything to you."

The night nurse gazed at me a moment. "Perhaps you're right," she said. "Perhaps empathy isn't possible without personal suffering." She paused and then added, "My husband had cancer. I nursed him."

I could feel our bond growing. "I wondered what made you so special."

*   *   *

In the morning I woke with a burst of optimism that the tubes would soon be removed and I'd be well enough to go home. Friends streamed in. I felt pampered. Friday was passing quickly. Rex arrived after work with homemade cards from Renae and Neil and a note from Kris. He went to the snack shop for a sandwich. I ripped open Kris's letter.

Stories of domestic squabbles prefaced the main issue. Kris had overheard someone say that I was foolish to leave the children with her, who they called "a drinker." Kris assured me that she hadn't had a drink since I left for the hospital. The tone of her note reminded me of her extraordinary potential for life. She was personable, adaptable, intelligent and sensitively witty. Previously, I had tried to convince Kris that people were trying to help at the house because of our friendship, not because they didn't trust her competence. That bit of overheard gossip had nullified my careful assurances. I was furious that anyone would have the insensitivity to label someone we loved by a problem of her past.

Certainly one of the most serious diseases of mankind is this tendency to summarize a person in a phrase.

I had feared the effect of gossip on our little ones. I hadn't realized Kris would also be vulnerable. I wanted to grab my clothes and rush home.

Rex returned from the snack shop. Before I could tell him my worries about Kris, Dr. Coulter, accompanied by a nurse, walked in and pulled the striped curtain to separate my half of the room from my roommate's. His first words were fantastic news. Because of my progress, he was ordering the discontinuation of intravenous fluids and the catheter. I almost cheered. My problems were solved. I'd soon be home to take care of my children and Kris.

But the way the doctor hesitated, I realized he wasn't finished. I joked, "What is this? The old good news, bad news routine?"

The nurse's averted face and Dr. Coulter's deliberate gaze told me that I had hit upon the truth. Consciously straightforward, Dr. Coulter went on. "Unfortunately you wasted your concern that a mastectomy might be unnecessary surgery. The lab report showed that there was lymph node involvement. I didn't discuss the report with you last night because I wanted to introduce your case to the tumor board, a group of surgeons which convenes every Friday morning to discuss treatment of new cancer patients."

I felt as if I had previously played this role. I remembered my part. As I had done after my outpatient surgery, I stared into the doctor's eyes. Again it seemed imperative that I remain outwardly calm and in control as I asked, "Didn't you say that my chances of survival would decrease from 95% to 45% if there was lymph-node involvement?"

"Yes, I did mention those statistics. But the best cure rates in women with node involvement are in the group with just one to three nodes involved. Out of seventeen nodes tested, only one of yours was affected. The infiltration of the lymph system is in an early stage."

At his side, the nurse nodded her head vigorously in agreement. Rex stood stunned, almost catatonic. The doctor placidly continued, "The lab reports also reveal that yours is an estrogen-dependent tumor."

Rex stirred. "What does that mean?" he asked.

"That means that Janet's cancer cells need estrogen to continue reproducing. That is very good news."

"Why?" Rex asked. "What do you do next?"

The tumor board agreed unanimously that we must remove the ovaries as soon as possible. The recent consensus in medical circles is that if a given tumor is estrogen dependent, removal of the source of estrogen logically should retard or eliminate the cancer's growth."

"So you want to remove her ovaries." Rex seemed to be having difficulty grasping the conversation. He moved in slow motion.

"You weren't planning to have more children, were you?" the doctor asked.

"No," we answered together.

"Then there's no disadvantage to the surgery. You'll just go through menopause ahead of your friends."

I wanted to run home and lock myself in my bedroom. Instead I asked, "When do you want to do the surgery?"

"Before you leave the hospital," he suggested. "You're already here and it's hard to come back. You will have to stay only about three days extra. As long as the uterus is healthy, which I expect it to be, the surgery is very simple."

"That doesn't sound too bad. Can you schedule me for tomorrow? I want to get home."

He laughed. "Not that soon. Your body needs a little time. We'll shoot for Tuesday. That's a week after your mastectomy. We'll plan to give you another unit of blood then. I think that would solve your problem of dizziness. We might as well wait until you're under anesthetic to give you the transfusion, though."

I was swept with gratitude at avoiding this extra pain.

The nurse brushed a tear from her face. I thought, We're just new friends and she's a veteran nurse. But she cares. How can she stand the emotional turmoil of this job? While I was observing her, Dr. Coulter turned and ordered, "Get rid of the I.V. and catheter immediately," and then he swiveled to leave.

Rex followed the doctor down the hall while the nurse re-moved the tubes. Now unencumbered except for the hemovac, I asked her, "Could I try one round with just Rex and smelling salts? I'm doing well tonight."

She understood.

I felt like a grand lady being escorted to a presidential ball as I shuffled in my white surgical stockings beside my man. When we returned I asked to sit in a chair for a while, but the effort of re-maining upright was exhausting. I submitted to being helped into the bed. Rex settled me and sat beside me, gently stroking the marks where the I.V. needle had been. "I guess we should have known that this whole thing couldn't be simple," he said.

I nodded. "I had hoped the mastectomy would be the end of it."

The nurses stopped to chat several times that evening—their presence an obvious offering of emotional support. One asked, "Are you doing all right?"

"Of course," I answered. Above all I would maintain the aura of coping. I refused to dissolve at the adverse news. It was as if I sat back viewing my own reactions. I simply stated, "I wish the report had been negative."

When I was alone that night, I thought, "Well, Father, I know you already know my condition."

"Yes, my child."

"Give me the strength to meet each day."

"I have promised that."

"Use me. Give me the strength to do the work you have for me each day that you give me."

"I have created you for good works."

"I'm tired."

"Come unto me, all ye who are heavy laden, and I will give you rest!"

"I'm afraid."

"Perfect love casts out fear."

"What happens next?"

"Whatsoever things are good . . ."

"Who will raise my children?"

"Whatsoever things are pure . . ."

"Will Rex sleep with another woman in our bed if I die?"

"Whatsoever things . . ."

"I know that four out of ten survive."

"Think on these things," God insisted.

"But how can I do that?"

"Remember my truths. You can do all things through me. I give you the strength and the power."

"But Father, I can't seem to focus my eyes to read your Word."

"That is why I told you to hide the Word in your heart. You are prepared."

And I quoted, "Peace I leave with you. Peace I give unto you. Not as the world gives, give I . . ."

Another Surgery

☙❧☙

"DR. COULTER, CALL 516. DR. COULTER, 516." THE PAGING SYSTEM woke me early Saturday morning. Since the previous Sunday, when I entered the hospital, I had observed that Dr. Coulter, a busy surgeon in a small hospital, was called more than any other doctor. But that Saturday I became obsessed with his name. I thought of the night before, as he stood at the foot of my bed stoically informing me of the spread of my cancer. I tried to imagine this day-and-night routine of dealing with life-and-death decisions. The strain of intricate surgery and responsible diagnosis —no wonder the number of general surgeons is relatively few. And no wonder Rex's and my intense questioning after out-patient surgery was disconcerting to him.

The warmth I felt for my doctor grew through the day. This was the man who was determining my future. Again I would have to lie physically naked before him. Emotionally, too, I felt stripped in front of him. I would submit to lying unconscious under his knife. I had to have explicit trust in his decisions and in his skill. I began to understand the fascination with soap operas such as "General Hospital." The intimacy between doctor and patient is certainly unmatched.

To me Dr. Coulter became a father figure. I loved this man who could deal with numerous crises and still treat me like a person. I wondered about his wife and children. I wondered how he had time for them. As the paging continued, I wondered how many meals had dried out while his wife waited for him to return from an unexpected dash to the hospital. After he sat kindly by my bed as if he had unlimited time for me, did he rush home and ignore his wife because he knew she understood? I surely wouldn't trade the life of a trucker's wife for that of a surgeon's, I thought.

Saturday night the doctor arrived late for his evening rounds. "Tomorrow I'm going to look at that leg," he commented about the dressing on the graft site. Apprehension must have shown on my face. "Oh, well," he went on, "why wait? I'm curious." And before I had a chance to suck in my breath, he had ripped the tape and it was over. He had saved me hours of dread. "It's healing nicely," he said. "We'll just leave that open to the air."

The next morning while Genny watched over me so that Mom could go to church, Dr. Coulter repeated his surprise tactics. This time while we were discussing his singing bass in the choir he turned and unexpectedly ripped the tape from the incision that extended under my arm and then, fraction by fraction, inched up a corner of the dressing. "Mmm! Doing fine. . . . It's time now for these tubes to come out." He motioned to the drainage tubes attached to the hemovac.

The rest of the conversation was a blur. I concentrated on hiding my panic.

The nurse who had been taking notes by his side returned and, almost timidly, approached the hemovac. Genny, my friend, my guardian angel, did not leave me. Quietly, firmly, she encouraged the nurse and the assistant to work as quickly as possible. To avoid the terror of the unknown I stared into Genny's familiar face. Dimly, I was aware of a vague sensation, perhaps as one can tell a tooth is being pulled even though the mouth is deadened by Novocain. I felt detached from my body. I viewed the events as they were reflected on Genny's face.

The staff nurses moved away from the bed. Genny smiled at me. "Are they finished? Is it over?" I asked.

The staff nurses left. My protection remained. "I couldn't have stood that if you hadn't been here to watch over me, Genny."

Sarah, the strong practical nurse who loved a challenge, returned almost immediately with a basin and a stack of towels. "How would you like your hair washed?" she asked.

I envisioned my clinging fear swirling down a drain with the suds. I was grateful to her for her insight.

* * *

Six days after my mastectomy, the morning before my second surgery, Rex's mother, Wanda, arrived from Florida. I had not seen her for the last three years. Phone calls do not replace visits. We held a marathon conversation. At one point I leaned back to rest and told her, "You know, I told Rex if you didn't have time to visit us when I was well, I didn't want you to come when I was sick and wouldn't be able to enjoy a visit. But I'm glad you didn't agree."

There were so many things I wanted Rex's mother to understand about Rex's adult personality. I wanted her to hear how diplomatically he had handled our first foster daughter. I wanted her to know that he was the one who had insisted on taking her in and that he maintained a patience in that year and a half that rivaled any saint's. I wanted her to know how he valued our own two little ones. How when offered a job that meant big money but separation from them for long periods of time, he chose the children, saying, "I can always make my fortune later." I wanted her to understand that Rex was a sensitive, caring adult—that most of the time he dropped his disguise of gruff harshness. "The nurses think I'm the luckiest woman in the world. Rex has won all their hearts with his boyish charm. They think he adores me. And so do I."

After work Rex popped in carrying several pieces of mail. He gave his mother and me both a kiss and announced that it was his turn to talk. "Look at this, Mom. All A's." He flourished a copy of my grades from graduate school. Rex had never boasted about my grades before. "Did you ever see such a thing?"

Slightly embarrassed, I tried to change the subject. "What else was in the mail?"

Rex turned accusingly. "Talking about mail. You never filled out the rest of those forms for Outstanding Young Women of America, did you?" He explained to his mother, "Several weeks ago she got a notice that she had been nominated for a book like *Who's Who*. Well, she had to send biographical information. I found this request for the information unanswered."

"It's nice to be considered, but those books are just money-making schemes. Who do you think buy the books? The people whose names are in it and their friends and relatives."

He ignored my comments. "I brought the papers with me because we're going to fill them out tonight." He did not deign to argue but matter-of-factly settled himself and declared, "I'll write and you talk." He began asking for dates and details. I didn't argue further. I was amused at Rex's new pride in everything I did, and I understood. He was afraid he was going to lose me. He now cherished my every act.

I dozed off as soon as Rex and I were alone. The doctor dropped in when I was sleeping. He woke me. "I heard that you were entertaining all day."

"Yes, I guess I did have a lot of friends stop by. And Rex's mother is here from Florida. We had a lot of catching up to do."

"I brought forms for you and Rex to sign. You'll notice that the permit for surgery is for an oophorectomy, an appendectomy and a hysterectomy. Removal of the ovaries is all that's necessary to stop hormone production and the incision for this procedure is quite small. But I need your permission to do the hysterectomy now in case I find problems with the uterus. I wouldn't want to wait and operate another time. If the uterus is healthy, though, we'll avoid the hysterectomy and speed up your recovery time." He parted by saying, "Get plenty of rest for our date tomorrow."

A nurse, Judy, returned to shave my abdominal and pubic area for surgery; she joked about my being skinny. She then reviewed the customary pre-op instructions and demonstrated the Try-flow, the little cage with three balls which registers different levels as you suck in—a game designed to encourage deep breathing after surgery so that the lungs won't fill with fluid. In preparation for the next day, I had to practice deep breathing and coughing, even though I winced in pain.

When Rex left, I asked Judy to help me arrange all the flowers in my room. I wanted all the wilted ones thrown away. I did not want to lie and watch them die. Then in privacy I took time to reread several notes from friends.

Our friend Ron, the one who had just separated from his wife, had tucked an insightful note to Rex in a get-well card:

Ann called last night to say that Janet needed more surgery and follow-up treatments. I wish I knew what to say that could be comforting to you both. Ann was in the hospital for a hyster-ectomy after Susie was born. She was sick and as usual I was busy and only made it over about once or twice in a week's time. To get to the point—Ann needed me and I did not make myself available to her.

Even though Janet may seem to be sick or in pain or tired, she will want you to be near as much as possible. You have a very good marriage and a love of the Lord so be thankful for that. This certainly is your greatest strength at this period of your lives.

I guess I am saying give Janet what she needs most right now—you. And I know that you have and that you will.

Yes, the love of my husband, my friends and my heavenly Father were my strength.

*   *   *

It seemed as if I had just fallen asleep when a nurse with a flashlight woke me. She lowered the side-rail and escorted me the few steps to the rest room. I wobbled across the floor like a Weeble in danger of falling down.

She brought out a catheter. I moaned. "I was just getting used to moving without tubes. Why do I have to have that again?"

"It's routine when surgery is in the abdominal area."
I submitted. "I'll be glad to get this over with."
I dozed. Our minister, Harry, woke me.
"You didn't have to come," I protested.
"I wanted to." He reassured me that Rex and the children were handling my hospitalization well. A militant nurse arrived to dismiss him. Harry used his ministerial voice. Mellowly and intensely he requested, "Could we have just a few more minutes?"
Like a geisha girl, she backed out. I loved her reaction. "Ministers must have power around here," I said.
"I've never been denied time yet."
"Maybe they think that you're administering the last rites."
We laughed. Harry shared my sense of humor.
The nurse returned to give me another pre-op injection. Feeling like a veteran of hospital procedure, I glibly answered her questions. "No, no dentures. No jewelry. No fingernail polish or contact lenses. Yes, please tape my wedding band." (I needed to take part of Rex with me on this ordeal.) I was slid onto a gurney to be transported to the operating room.
Harry returned, followed by my entourage—Rex, Wanda and three other friends. The elevator groaned as my fans squeezed tightly against the walls around me. We were as silly as a crowd at a Mardi Gras festival. The aide halted the procession at the lounge door. "You will all have to stay here," she gestured. "The doctor will be out to talk to you after surgery," she said to Rex.
My cheerful aide announced me to the operating room staff. As she turned to leave, I naively said, "I'll see you shortly. This should be a cinch."
As the doors swished closed behind the aide, I turned my eyes and saw that an anesthetist had arrived and was reading my chart. The anteroom was empty. This time it appeared that there would be no waiting.
"I'm Janet Britton," I introduced myself as he reached automatically for my wrist band.
He glanced at my name and returned to the chart. "Ah, yes, Janet Britton—bilateral oophorectomy and appendectomy."
"Yes, hopefully that's all. Are you having a slow day down here?"

For the first time he looked me in the face. "We're right on schedule for a change," he said, grinning.

"I'm glad. A person could get nervous waiting out here."

A flowered attendant arrived. "Janet Britton?" she asked. I giggled. The irony of the scene struck me. These people who held life and death in their hands were dressed absurdly. Their blue-and-green flowered gowns reminded me of my mother in her flannel pajamas and nightcap, without the lace trim, of course.

A mute attendant wheeled me to the operating room—the land of backs and eyelids. My arrival was unheralded, but an automatic sensor must have warned the workers. A metallic voice was switched on as flowered gowns moved toward my gurney. "Slide onto the table, please."

Awkwardly I struggled to propel my leaden body. My bare back slid onto an icy slab. The jolt to my left side woke the pain that had been lulled by the hypos. A robot hand reached for my left arm. "Please don't stretch that arm. I just had surgery last week. I'm sore."

A flicker of lids registered awareness of my pain. The robot's control panel shifted down the gears and its speed decreased.

I tried to reach behind the steel shells to the humans who hid behind them. "Don't you freeze working in here?" I smiled ingratiatingly. The attendant positioning shiny instruments soon to be smeared with my blood shrugged, untouched.

I turned my head to the right side and repeated my question. Raising brown lids, the anesthetist peaked out from behind his automaton's face. Shyly, he responded, "You get used to it." I was grateful for a glimpse of his humanity.

Dr. Coulter arrived. His eyes brushed mine.

"I hope we don't keep meeting like this," I joked.

His eyes laughed. He answered, "This should take care of everything."

"You are going to go to sleep now," the anesthetist intoned, safely sheltered once more behind his brown lids. "Count backward from 100."

Passively, I obeyed. "Ninety-nine, ninety-eight, ninety-seven, ninety—"

*   *   *

The chart at the nurse's station recorded that I returned from the recovery room to room 321 at 12:45, although dim sensory impressions were my only record of that Tuesday's events. While I was in the recovery room, occasionally a spectral creature floated into my gray hazy world. I strained to see the vague apparitions who hovered in and out of my sphere, but the lens on my vision's camera would not respond to my weak commands.

On the trip to my room, I became an acrobat balancing a board atop a giant ball. The motion stopped. I floated across a ravine to my hospital bed. Foreign ghost images were joined by hazy replicas of familiar people—Rex, Mom, Wanda. But their faces were distorted into gargoyle expressions. I strained to see their features clearly, but it was like trying to view a drive-in picture screen in a fog. Voices echoed across a chasm. I attempted to focus. My eyes acted like a zoom camera lens focusing in close and then out far away. I could not control the zoom lens.

I felt pressure on my chin and became aware that I was vomiting. Pain from the strain of heaving shot through my chest and abdomen. Rex held the kidney-shaped bowl under my mouth, but his hand evidently shook for the bowl seemed to dart away from me.

I froze. I shook. The weight of a pile of blankets pressed on me but did not insulate me. I continued to freeze as the pile heightened.

I heaved and heaved. The liquid stopped. My heaving continued. A nurse arrived. She jabbed my hip. My heaving stopped. I whirled in a cloud of nausea. I floated on the gas which inflated my abdomen. I belched, but the gas continued to expand. I feared floating around the room like a helium balloon. I feared a nurse's syringe would explode me.

Seemingly, months passed while I resided in the Land of Pain. I floated aimlessly, without anchor or propulsion, living in a dimension without time—a dimension of sensation, pain, nausea, drifting, falling, swirling, straining to return. Aware only of being cradled in my Father's arms, I remembered, "Peace I give unto you, not as the world gives, give I." Should I stay with my Father and rest or should I return to my worldly home and work? I really had no choice—I remained trapped in a body of pain. The tapes in my mind played "Great Is Thy Faithfulness." The world of time knocked, shifting me to one side and poking my hips, probing under my tongue, tightening bands on my arm, commanding me to breathe deeply.

* * *

And then, shockingly, I was catapulted permanently into the world of time. As if smelling salts had been waved under my nose, I woke clearly to a wave of nausea accompanying the smell of bacon and coffee. It was Wednesday morning, the day after my surgery. The cover had been lifted from my roommate's breakfast tray. I tried to control the swirling world.

Water nauseated me. I attempted sips of juice, of ginger ale—nausea. I slaked my thirst by running ice chips across my lips.

"I have to eat," I insisted, but my body wouldn't cooperate.

I buzzed for a nurse. "I need to walk when you have the time to escort me." As I walked, the pain in my abdomen increased. But the transfusion had helped. Although I was faint, I didn't pass out.

"That wasn't too bad," I puffed as I eased myself back down. The nurses adjusted me into a freshly made bed. I stared at the wall and hummed softly under my breath, attempting to force air out to control my belching. Time drifted.

Gas swelled my abdomen. Visitors streamed in and out of my room. I responded to their conversations with the robotlike detachment of the operating room staff. Evening came. I leaned back, making no attempt to talk as three friends snickered over the rowdy hillbilly family visiting in the next room. These friends would accept, without dramatic relaying of my condition, my need to rest.

Dozing momentarily in the peaceful contentment of friendship, I was startled by a rending cry in the hall. I jerked my head to see what catastrophe had occurred. To my shock, there stood Rex's distant cousin, Gert, sobbing, "Oh Janet, I'm so sorry." The scene seemed cut from a 1930s melodrama. Gert, dressed in a purple print dress, leaned on a walking stick with one hand and clutched Cousin Andy's arm with the other. Rivulets flowed from her clenched eyes. Andy futilely tried to console her while balancing a huge vase of flowers. He managed to steer Gert into the room and wedge her into a chair. Whenever she sucked in a breath, the wailing was replaced by a faint whine like that of a jet engine. I tried to make her hear. "I'm just fine. Really I am. I'll be out of here soon. I'm just fine."

I forced my eyes wide open, hoping to look soon-to-be-healthy. Rex bore the load of the conversation. I tried not to burp. I tried not to swallow air. I felt as if I were being pumped up with a bicycle pump. It seemed as if years were passing. Gert, like a mountain, loomed immovable. I feared she had laid siege to my room. Several times Rex discreetly offered to walk Andy and Gert to the elevator, but they ignored him. Ages later, with a final mournful shake of her head, Gert lumbered into the hall.

My other visitors had sat transfixed through this ordeal. "You must be awfully close to them," one observed.

In spite of my discomfort, I started to chuckle. "Let me give you a clue. They live twelve miles away, and we haven't seen them for two years. We probably haven't seen them more than five times in thirteen years of marriage. I have no idea, even, how they learned I was in the hospital."

Our suppressed giggles were interrupted by the announcement that visiting hours were over. As everyone rose to leave, I begged Rex to stay a little longer to walk me in the hall, because one of the nurses had told me that walking encourages peristalsis, the normal bowel action which relieves gas.

As Rex helped me sit up, I winced. "My stomach feels like it's on fire."

We walked the hall. On the right side, past the nurses' kitchen. Past the storage room. Past the drinking fountain. Past the lounge. Past the elevator. Past the elegant lady with two black eyes and a leg in traction. We turned and, on the opposite side of the hall, shuffled past the "isolation" notice and past the old man strapped to his chair. We paused to exchange comments with the eighteen-year-old boy who was injured on a motorcycle. We turned at the nurses' station. We passed the diabetes patient who had just had her leg amputated. We passed the muffled moan of the woman in the room beside mine. We passed my roommate, who smiled. And then again we walked past the nurses' kitchen. Past the storage room. . . .

"This time we'll stop at your room," urged Rex.

"I don't feel any better."

"You're exhausted."

"Sitting won't help. Only walking."

"You should rest. Don't overdo." He paused, almost shyly. "I love you."

I leaned contentedly on his shoulder, oblivious of onlookers. Then I forced myself to forge ahead. Repeatedly, we retraced our path.

After several hours I admitted defeat and sent Rex home. As the nurse, Judy, helped me into bed, I warned her not to touch my stomach because even the brushing of the sheet made my skin feel as if thousands of tiny pins were pricking it. She saw the tautness of my skin and buzzed for another nurse. Judy explained her concern. "I prepped her for surgery and her abdomen was flat—concave actually. Now look at her."

They listened for bowel sounds and left. My pain increased. With a combination of professional and personal reassurance, they returned to tell me that Dr. Coulter would be in soon to check me.

I could no longer push back the fear that something had gone wrong in surgery. Nightmarish thoughts of a missing instrument floating in my body or of sutures that had ruptured swarmed in my mind. I couldn't repress the fear that I was too weak to go under anesthetic again.

A lab technician flew in to do a "Complete Blood Count—Stat." Nurses from the midnight shift, Ruth and Amy, wheeled in an I.V. unit ("The doctor wants a glucose started before he gets here") and instructed me to "pump your arm. Clench your fist." They tapped my arm repeatedly as they looked for a needle site. Both nurses shook their heads and decided it would be best to call the I.V. team. I concentrated on deep breathing to try to relax.

Then Amy and Ruth were replaced by strangers, an I.V. therapist and the nursing supervisor, who ignored me as if I were a piece of metal being molded in a factory. "These young nurses always overreact. From what I hear, all she needs is a little rest. She's had too much company."

The I.V. therapist, searching for a vein, smacked my hand and arm. After several minutes she straightened up, arched her back, and then leaned over again and disgustedly barked, "No wonder we can't get the needle in. Her arm's as stiff as a board."

Every nerve of my body felt exposed, and she had the audacity to criticize me for being tense. Mimicking her tone, I snapped, "Just ask me to relax it then."

Both swiveled their heads—in disbelief, apparently, that metal can speak.

Time crawled by. At last Dr. Coulter strode in, exuding confidence. I apologized for disturbing his sleep.

Smiling, he instructed me, "I'm going to insert this tube down your nose. Swallow." I had no choice. It was either swallow or choke to death. I gagged and gulped as the tube was slid down my nose into my stomach to pump. He continued talking. "I can usually wake up alert even if I've been sleeping soundly. Except for the other night. I answered the phone right after I had dozed off. I was in that deep sleep right at the beginning of the night."

I nodded, gasping.

"Someone described his symptoms, and I told him to meet me in a half-hour and I'd give him some medication. I hung up. And then I realized that I hadn't told him where to meet me, and I couldn't remember who I'd talked to." He chuckled. "I waited and waited by my office. Finally I took the medicine to the hospital emergency room, figuring that eventually he'd end up there asking for me. I felt a little strange telling the nurse I was expecting a patient but didn't know who it would be."

His story was an obvious effort to get my mind off the pain. It worked.

But he was interrupted by the I.V. therapist. "We're still looking for a vein."

"Well, you have to find one," the doctor insisted. "We'll use the left arm if we have to."

Oh, please, Lord. Let them find a vein in my right arm.
At last—success.

The nurse handed the doctor a rubber glove, and he inserted a rectal suppository. After submitting me to this final indignity, he told me to rest and started to leave. A floor nurse stopped him to suggest that he restrict visitors to the immediate family. Ruth returned with another hypo. I lay with green fluid pumping from my nose. My taut skin began to relax.

Time drifted in and out of the pain. I viewed the room from the wrong end of a telescope. I was a tightrope walker on a wire stretched over a great canyon. Every muscle strained.

Listening to the muffled night sounds of the hospital, I used my newly developed techniques to try to lull myself to sleep. I forced myself to lie without stirring, eyes riveted to the light at the tip of the nurses' buzzer, hoping that sleep would sneak up surreptitiously. Since counting lambs jumping over a fence was too conventional, mentally I stared at a "Sesame Street" screen as numbers to teach counting were flashed one at a time. Each digit received equal billing. When I reached 1,000, I started over. I set 5,000 as my limit. But I was still awake, so softly I sang— "The Lord's Prayer," "Great Is Thy Faithfulness," "One Day at a Time." My repertoire was limited. I knew melodies to hundreds of songs, but as a pianist I had ignored lyrics. All my methods failed to induce sleep, though. As dawn broke, I admitted defeat —moments before I drifted away.

* * *

Nausea, dizziness, acrid ammonia capsules, pain, chills, fever —the sensations of the next days blended together. Mom and Wanda alternated between finding more blankets to cover me and wiping the sweat from my face and neck with cool washcloths. I found Sir Thomas Wyatt's line running through my mind: "I burn, and freeze like ice."

Rex insisted that the thermostat on the air-conditioning unit in the window next to my bed be fixed. Once the room temperature was regulated more precisely, I wished the maintenance man would stay and fix my body's thermostat. I was not living in the comfort of my once-familiar body. I had moved from my former body with its gas furnace kept comfortably at 68 degrees to a body with a coal furnace which first blasted me with scorching air and then cooled until I shivered and stoked the fire again.

In the quiet produced by the "No Visitors" sign on my door, I dozed fitfully day and night. The changing of the guard—Mom, Wanda, Rex—occurred so quietly, so smoothly, that often I was unaware for hours that there had been a change.

Often I woke and found the curtain between my roommate and me closed and the window curtains drawn. Stripes, not a rainbow, but a prison. "Please don't close me in. I want to see what's happening."

"You need your rest," Mom urged.

"I can't stand the curtains. Push them back."

Later I'd wake and find the curtains pulled once again. The flowers' perfume made me feel like the corpse in a funeral home. I couldn't explain this reaction to my mother. So, irritably, I fussed. "It's one thing to be stuck in this bed. Don't make me feel as if I'm locked in. I have to see the world."

I asked about the children. I was too tired to dwell on the answers. Too tired to talk to them on the phone. Too tired even to worry.

I was too tired to talk to Rex. Too tired to pray to God. Both understood. Both reached through the tubes and held me.

Since I could not comfortably hold a Bible even if I had had energy to read one, I understood the importance of "hiding the Word in my heart."

"What time I am afraid, I will trust in thee." "I have learned, in whatsoever state I am, therewith to be content." "I can do all things through Christ who strengthens me."

Nervously, I listened for the warning buzzer on the I.V. My hand and arm ached. "How does your arm feel?" the I.V. therapist asked. "Just fine," I lied, hoping the site would not be moved.

I prayed to pass gas. I understood the passage in 1 Corinthians about the body of Christ and how important the uncomely parts are to the functioning of the church. Previously unable even to define the term *peristalsis,* I had always taken my intestines' function for granted—I had even been embarrassed by their existence. And now the attention of the hospital staff and each of my family members was centered on my bowels; everyone's first question was whether I had passed gas yet. None of the "comely" members of my body could work if an unmentionable part didn't do its role. The comparison of the body to the church family took on new meaning.

At last on Friday evening, I forced out the tiniest little air bubble. I called to Rex, "Peristalsis has begun!" We celebrated as we had at the first steps of each of the children.

"I'm going to thank the Lord every day for peristalsis," I promised Rex. "Don't ever let me forget."

When the doctor made his evening rounds several hours later, I feigned vigorous health. My efforts were rewarded. "I think we can remove your tubes now. You'll be home in a few days."

I rejoiced. Freedom from the I.V. Freedom from the catheter. Freedom from the stomach tube. And the promise of eventual freedom from my hospital bed. Soon I would be an independent entity once again.

"Take your wife for a walk," I urged Rex when the doctor left. Joyfully I held his arm as he escorted me down the aisle once more.

*   *   *

A new nurse, brassy and obese, arrived with Saturday's morning shift. Her voice reverberated in my head as she proceeded to cheer up the patients with her textbook phrases. "Rise and shine. Let's get washed up."

Susan, a nurse friend, brushed past her and helped me to the bathroom. I sponged up by myself, consciously controlling my dry heaves and dragged myself to my bed and slumped back weakly. Abruptly I was catapulted upright by the jet-propelled cranking of the head of my bed. It was the new nurse. "Is this about right?" she asked. Before I could reposition the stomach that had been thrust into my mouth, she banged my tray on the bedstand, whirled it in front of me, launched the cover from the plates and commanded, "Eat it all up." Grape juice, cherry Jell-O and tea—

my liquid diet. I wondered how many flavors of gelatin there are.

The new nurse, accompanied by an aide, then deposited me in a chair while they changed the sheets. My stare fixed on the raveled edges of her uniform sleeves and the greasy roots of her frizzed hair. "No," I thought. "Whatsoever things are good . . ."

I asked about the portrait necklace dangling from her neck. "Whose babies are those?"

She glowed. "Mine! They're five-month-old twins."

"You must hate leaving them to come to work."

"Oh, I only work one weekend a month. Just enough to give me a break from the babies—a little time out of the house."

The doctor, wearing his rolled green pants for surgery, dashed into the room. Checking my incisions, he mumbled something about changing my dressing. As he spoke, he loosened the tape from the center top corner. Rapidly and gently it was done. I sighed in relief.

Trotting on his way, smiling at his own skill, he ordered my care. "I want the graft area washed with a Betadine solution and a four-by-four fluff dressing applied twice a day." Moments later the brassy one flopped back in, bandages and tape in hand. I stopped her. "Could Susan do my dressing, please?"

"I don't see what difference it makes." She ignored me, starting to rip off the rest of the tape.

I didn't want this cold stranger to stare at my missing breast. I sensed, or perhaps imagined, her curiosity about this mastectomy. I wanted a nurse who saw Janet and not a grotesque disfigurement. But, too, I wanted to be known as an intelligent adult, not a neurotic mastectomy patient. I steeled myself. I would not show her how much I dreaded this. I submitted without further comment, staring at the curtain that separated me from the world.

"Oh, I see you had quite a large graft." I ignored her attempt to make conversation. "You seem upset. How do you feel about your surgery?" I could not speak. I could not trust my voice to be steady. "It's important for you to deal with your emotions. Would you like to talk about your feelings to me?" No, not to an insensitive stranger.

The doctor had moved swiftly but gently. This nurse worked as if she were wearing boxing gloves. I tried to detach myself from the scene. She continued to prod. "You ought to cry. You would feel much better if you'd just cry."

I broke down and spoke. "Crying makes me feel miserable."

"It's not healthy to deny your emotions."

"It's not healthy for me to let myself go."

She squirted Betadine solution and spread it with sterile gauze. I was shocked. I dreaded antiseptic solution on my wound because I anticipated pain. But I felt nothing. Somewhere in my brain I recorded an awareness of being touched. But I was numb, a block of wood. Not only had I lost the body of a woman, I had also lost the sensations of a human being.

"What are you thinking? Tell me what you feel about your surgery." Again she beat on my weak defenses. My thin shield against emotional collapse cracked and tears trickled through, turning into hot rivers running unchecked down my cheeks, onto my neck and onto the crisp white pillowcase.

"It's so degrading," I sniffled.

"Why do you say that? What is degrading?"

"You wouldn't understand," I sobbed, unable to stop the cascade of tears. I was angry. I was embarrassed. I felt as exposed as if I had walked naked into my classroom of senior English students. "Just hurry and finish what you have to do," I croaked and turned my face. I swallowed, trying to breathe more slowly. But the crack in the dike had ruptured. The flood would not stop. I had been defeated in my attempt to maintain my dignity.

The rotund one, collecting the supplies, cheerfully clucked, "You'll feel better now that you've had a good cry."

I did not respond.

Finally she vacated the room. Mom slipped back in. Without comment, she took a brush and arranged my hair off my forehead. I whimpered, "I'm so angry. I fell to pieces."

"Don't worry about it. You know your hormones are out of balance."

I couldn't help smiling. Mom's explanation for all our mysterious depressions, ever since I was twelve years old, was, "Don't worry. It's probably your hormones." I paused, waiting for the traditional lines to follow. "Go ahead and cry. Tears wash your eyes and make them sparkle." Mom's familiar phrases soothed me. That same advice had accompanied every cut knee, every skinned elbow, every disappointment and broken heart.

Susan glided in and I burst out, "I wanted you to change my dressing. I wanted a friend."

"I tried to stop her," Susan apologized. "I said I'd be glad to do the dressing change but she insisted."

"Did I have the right to refuse to let her touch me? I didn't want to raise a fuss and make problems for you."

Susan assured me that no nurse could administer treatment without the patient's consent. She promised to change my dressing every day she was on duty. I was relieved by that thought, but I couldn't forget the other nurse.

"She didn't understand, did she?" I asked Mom and Susan. "I need to be brave—not for other people, but for me."

* * *

Mom guarded me. I dozed. Lunch trays woke me. Bouillon and lime Jell-O and tea. In my assertive mood I demanded that Mom find me some crackers. She hesitated, but I was determined. When the doctor arrived, about four o'clock that afternoon, I was prepared to argue. Tersely I pointed out that anybody would be nauseated who had to live on bouillon and Jell-O. If I was going to get better, I needed food. He chuckled and ordered the nurse, "Get her a tray."

"Change her to a soft diet?"

I shook my head, pleading, and he laughed. "Give her anything that sounds good to her." Stubbornly I choked down bites of potatoes, roast beef, peas and pudding—a banquet. I insisted to myself that I couldn't possibly be more nauseated than I had been on the liquid diet. And since I was going to burp anyway, I might as well taste something I enjoyed the first time. The resulting nausea seemed no more intense than it had been.

Then, thinking about coping with another dressing change, I lay with anxiety mounting until Rex arrived. "What if I'm tied up

in knots like this every day, waiting for my dressing changes?"
I asked him.

He squeezed my hand. "You just had a bad experience. It'll be
all right with Bobbi this evening. And on her days off Amy works.
On day shift Susan or Judy will take care of you. You'll be fine."

I wanted to believe him. He leaned over and further assured
me. "We've gone through a lot together. Don't worry. I'll sit with
you while Bobbi changes the bandage tonight."

Later Bobbi, one of our favorite nurses on the afternoon shift,
entered my room with her bandages, her Betadine, her scissors
and—most important—her smile and her sparkling eyes which
gazed deeply into mine.

"You don't mind an audience, do you?" Rex asked.

"Of course not."

"I was a big baby this afternoon," I told her.

"I've always liked to work in pediatrics," she joked.

Puzzled, Bobbi scrutinized my dressing. She trotted back to
the nurses' station for a copy of the doctor's orders. "Cover
wound with a four-by-four fluffed dressing," the orders read.

"Oh, she was to have opened the four-by-four dressing and
applied it loosely. That would make it almost an eight-by-eight.
Quite a difference, wouldn't you say?"

Deftly she began loosening the dressing. "I'll soak this with
Betadine solution to help unstick it. . . . There, that doesn't look
bad. It's healing nicely. Just that one corner of the graft is seeping
significantly. Janet, you don't need to worry about looking at
this."

My head began to swirl at the thought of looking at caked
pus and blood, and I suggested a change of topic. We three discussed my new flowers, the pile of cards I'd received that day,
Bobbi's boyfriend's new car. . . . The dressing change was completed. As Rex and Bobbi were helping me slip into a fresh gown,
Bobbi said, "At least you don't have to worry about stitches or
dressings on your abdominal incision." I peeked down at a silver
line, shiny like a teflon-coated ironing-board cover, clinging to
my pubic hairline. I had never heard of this surgical superglue.
I was grateful that at least that incision needed no care. Bobbi

stayed a few more minutes, making sure my psychological wounds were as comfortably bandaged as my physical ones were. I sighed. I had made it. With the help of a nurse friend and my lover, I didn't feel like "the mastectomy in room 321." I had been treated as a very precious individual—who just happened to have recently had surgery.

When Bobbi left the room, Rex leaned over and kissed my forehead. "I could never have made it without you," I said. "But I wish you hadn't had to see how ugly I am."

Rex gathered his words carefully. "You'll never be ugly to me. Actually, I'm glad I saw your chest now. When it's healed, I'll always remember how much better you are."

I loved Rex for many reasons. One of them was his total honesty. Another was his familiarity with my need for a verbal description. He was the one I cuddled against in those gory Clint Eastwood movies of our honeymoon year, my eyes hidden against his shoulder. He knew that as soon as the scene was over, I would ask, "What happened?" and expect a complete description. My mind could accept what my eyes could not.

He now described for my mind what my eyes rejected. "The part that looks worst is the skin graft. It runs at a diagonal and is purple and raw looking. It's the size of the mark on your leg—about four inches by two inches. The rest of your chest and up under your arm looks like any other stitches."

When my curiosity had been satisfied, I clung tightly to his hard brown fingers and said, "You're so good to me. You're the only person in the world I could trust to describe it to me honestly. I wish Bobbi understood why I won't look, though."

We leaned together, grateful that the hurdle had been cleared.

* * *

Sunday, August 31, a woman from Reach for Recovery was scheduled to visit me. Part of me appreciated this woman's willingness to take time to help a stranger. But I couldn't shake my cynical attitude toward all agency representatives. I summarized this negativism to my sister Bonnie. "I don't know if I'll be able to stand a sweet lady telling me how to cope."

From the moment the woman stepped into my room, though, her expression and her words struck me as genuine.

She brimmed with anecdotes: "My husband and I love to square dance. A friend of ours grabbed me under the arms on a 'swing your partner' and couldn't look me in the face for the rest of the night." She threw her head back and roared and then began another tale. "I went back to my office job before I had the chance to buy my prosthesis. So I just grabbed several of my husband's socks and stuffed them into my bra. Well anyway, everyone was a little nervous about my being back so soon. One of the maintenance men came in for a purchase order. He sort of just stared around the room. I thought it was a little unusual that he avoided looking directly at me, since we've been good friends for years. About ten minutes later I went to comb my hair and I about died. There one side of my chest was flat and I had a gigantic lump near my collarbone. My bra with its socks had slid up. All I could do at that point was double over laughing. It does help to have a sense of humor after a mastectomy!" Bonnie and I giggled with her as she entertained us with her stories.

She also brimmed over with practical information. Uninhibitedly she unbuttoned her blouse, handed me her prosthesis and showed me her flat white scar. In my hand, the artificial breast was huge and heavy. Returned to her bra, it hung as pendulous as her natural breast.

I grinned. "Mine will be a midget version of yours. In fact I think a padded bra would take care of me just fine."

But she strongly disagreed, stating that a weighted prosthesis would eliminate the need to secure one side of the bra to my undergarment. She advised me on postmastectomy fashions and demonstrated the best exercises for regaining full use of my left arm.

That afternoon was happily filled with visits from my loving family. I tried to imagine facing cancer alone and uninformed. I shut out the thought, but it led to an unquenchable urge to go home. As we trudged up and down the hall, Rex and I engineered a foolproof escape plan. "I'll duck into this storage room, and you can go back to the room and gather up my belongings,"

I began. Quickly, Rex caught the spirit of my fantasy.

"I'll borrow your Mom's trench coat, and we'll wrap up the rest of your nightgowns and robes and shove them under the coat. People will think you're a pregnant lady on a dry run to the hospital. That will also cover any suspicion aroused by your wearing slippers, because people will just think your feet are too swollen for your shoes."

"I'd better take off my surgical hose."

"Oh, people will assume white hose are the new attire for the fashionable lady-in-waiting." Rex mimicked a pregnant woman's waddle.

Laughing at him, I cautiously suggested that we formulate an emergency plan in case we were detected. "You know I can't run to elude the hounds."

"I'll drag you."

"I couldn't stand the pain from my incisions."

"I'll carry you piggyback."

"I don't have enough strength to hold onto your neck."

"We'll steal a wheelchair."

"Aha, that will work."

"Are you ready to leave now?"

I sighed. "Yes, I want to. But I'm so tired from all this planning that I think I should rest tonight. Tomorrow will be better. I'll escape then and we'll have a family Labor Day picnic."

Rex's blue eyes twinkled. I love his sense of humor, I thought. After thirteen years of marriage, I am still attracted to his light heart.

Gently Rex kissed my cheek. Affection in public, even, I marveled. My illness has been nothing but good for our relationship.

All day Sunday I floated on a cloud of love and optimism. I was cushioned by the emotional support of my family and by the hope that soon I could really "escape" to my normal life. That evening, though, my spirits sagged. By ten o'clock I had a fever and was belching profusely. The nurse had no answer when I asked her why I was feeling so ill. I couldn't shake my major concern: the doctor wouldn't let me out if I stayed dizzy and nauseated. And I missed my family so!

Chanting memory verses and humming hymns, at last I began my cycle of dozing and waking.

*   *   *

Monday, Labor Day, I woke to the second day of my third week in the hospital. While Rex and the children enjoyed a quiet morning at home, Mom and I spent the time leisurely rereading my cards and letters.

The stack of cards and letters from Ann and Ron, the couple who now lived separately in Virginia, convinced me of their continued friendship. I smiled as I retraced the events of my hospitalization through their references to phone conversations with Rex. In one note, Ron summed up our friendship: "We four have shared some very good times together and lately some traumatic times. No matter what, I will always cherish those times and hope we can all repeat them once again." For several minutes I reveled in memories of what we called the Bonner-Britton Corporation.

Loneliness for Ann and Ron made me treasure our other friends that much more. Nostalgic, I dialed several to keep ties tight. When I apologized that neither Rex nor I had called, one interrupted me gently. "We knew that when you were ready and well enough we'd have lots of time to talk. We really didn't need all the details to pray for you or to take your family a pie either."

Succinctly, she had summarized the position of my true friends.

Waking the next morning, Tuesday, I smiled at the memory of Genny's repeated messages to "Rest, relax and give your body a chance to heal." But today I needed to organize my students' classes. I had requested that the substitute be paid to spend an in-service day with me to discuss the programs. Today was the day for that scheduled meeting. I arranged to look my best so the sub would carry optimistic reports about me back to school. Before eight o'clock, a friend trotted in with her blow dryer and curling iron, according to plan. In a flash she whipped out shampoo and conditioner, a basin and towels and was ready to transform me.

"You should advertise," I joked. "Emergency beauty care—have brush, will travel."

By 9:15 I was dressed in my fluffy pink bed jacket, which hid my bandages. Carefully made up and coifed, I looked like a new woman.

Time tiptoed slowly by. Just when I had almost given up on the teacher's coming, she tripped in, babbling excuses for being so late. I sensed that she was anxious to dart away, so I launched right into the task by asking about her favorite books. "I don't have much time to read for pleasure," she told me. I had to restrain myself. I wanted to scream "Heresy!" and insist that she had to be an avid reader if she was to stimulate student interest in books.

"Do you like to teach writing?"

"Well, I don't feel very well prepared to teach composition. That's why I concentrate on grammar. If they know the rules, I figure they can write when they have to."

No, no, no, I refrained from shouting. People learn to write by writing—not by filling in one-word answers in grammar drills. I avoided getting on my soapbox, though; I suppressed my desire to lecture.

Mentally, I girded myself. A grammarian with no love for reading! This was going to be hard. But young and perhaps impressionable. Maybe she could be swayed to save time by using my methods instead of developing her own approach to the courses.

I had completed discussing the writing courses and had begun describing the format of the independent reading program when I caught Wanda's stare. I looked away from her concerned eyes. I forced eye contact with the substitute, hoping that if I was direct and professional she would catch my intensity. I felt like a marathon runner who had reached the wall. If I could just push on, I knew that somehow I would find the strength to finish.

And I did. The moment the substitute disappeared through the door, though, I slumped weakly over the right side of the chair. I longed to lie down but did not have the strength to move from the chair to the bed.

Wanda rushed to my side. "Janet, are you all right?"

"I feel as if I just taught six weeks of classes in two-and-a-half hours. It was impossible. Did I sound energetic? Did I sound convincing?" My eyes begged for positive feedback.

"You made sense to me," she reassured me as she hoisted me toward the bed.

My legs felt like sponge. I was limp all over. Wanda lifted my legs onto the bed and slipped a pillow under my head. I shook uncontrollably. No matter how hard I clenched my jaw, I could not stop the clattering of my teeth. Pain shot through my chest and abdomen as the shaking bed jarred my incisions. Wanda piled blankets on me and simultaneously rang for the nurse who rushed in with hot tea and an injection. A haze filled the room.

"How could you do such a dumb thing to yourself?" Wanda nervously scolded me.

"It's over now," I whispered. "And I did it. Now I won't have to worry about school anymore. I'll just get better."

*　*　*

In my third week in the hospital, I continued to refuse pain medication until Mom's or Rex's prodding insistence convinced me to yield. Emotionally I was governed by my father's reluctance to take any drug.

My father's early avoidance of medication was logical. Terminally ill, he knew that the pain would progressively worsen as days passed and that the future effectiveness of the medicine depended on his avoiding it as long as possible. But later, when the pain was excruciating, he found that if the medication clouded the pain, it also clouded his reasoning ability. So Dad continued to insist that narcotics be kept to a minimum. "If I'm unconscious, I might as well be dead already." Rationally I knew that our situations were different. But although there was no logic in refusing to be more comfortable until I healed from surgery, I still rebelled. I had a family tradition to uphold. I wouldn't be known as a "sniveler."

When I did submit, the hypo made me uptight. I couldn't decide if my reaction was chemical or psychological. I despised the floating "spaced-out" sensation that some of my students sought. Pain to me was at least a familiar reminder of my humanity. Like the savage in *Brave New World,* I loathed the artificial euphoria.

Inwardly I remained convinced that the way to get better was to fight every minute—fight the pain, fight the nausea and dizziness, and fight to keep moving. But finally after one particularly fitful night, I asked my surgeon if he would set aside some time to talk. Dr. Coulter, who had been paged at least ten times in three hours, had been in surgery all morning and was on his way to an office full of patients, settled himself onto my bed as if he were readying himself for an afternoon at the beach. "I have all the time in the world right now," he lied skillfully. For a moment, I believed him.

Immediately I launched into a tirade of how discouraged I was. I had understood that I'd only be in the hospital about three days after the oophorectomy, but a week had already passed, and obviously it was going to be even longer. "If you told me I needed to hang from the curtain rod three times a day, by my toes even, I'd figure some way to do it if you could explain logically how it would help. But sometimes I wonder if I'm concentrating on the wrong things."

Dr. Coulter listened patiently, deliberated a few minutes and then said, "Right now, I think there's nothing either of us can do to hurry the process of healing. Your body has had a shock." He went on to explain that recovery from the removal of ovaries is normally quick, because oophorectomies are usually done on older women whose estrogen level is already declining. Also, in younger women surgeons routinely implant a tablet of synthetic estrogen which dissolves over a period of months and allows the gradual tapering of hormone levels. But I had gone from peak production of estrogen to zero production. "I can't intervene. I can only observe and record your symptoms," he said, "because the purpose of the surgery was to stop estrogen production and retard the cancer."

I told him I still couldn't understand why I felt pregnant. I grinned. "Am I really expecting and you're afraid to tell me?"

Dr. Coulter's reserve melted. He threw his head back and laughed. "If you are, I'll take pictures of the delivery and we'll both be wealthy." He explained that my sensations were similar to pregnancy because both resulted from drastic hormone imbalances.

He paused. "Forget about going home for a while. Relax and take whatever time your body needs to regulate itself."

The doctor's attitude reinforced my family's urgings to accept pain medication so that I could be comfortable. It was Genny, though, who provided the final argument. "When you're fighting pain, you're tensing the injured tissues and interfering with their healing ability." From that time on, I accepted medication. I amused myself by playfully offering Rex my hips to play dot-to-dot games and by grading each nurse's injections.

In other ways, too, I started following my body's signals instead of fighting them. Since my nausea was most intense before noon, I slept as much as possible in the morning and exercised more in the afternoon and evening. Since even a sip of cool water nauseated me, I drank warmed ginger ale and the decaffeinated spice tea that Harry brought me. My mother, Wanda and Rex walked with me, brought crackers, made tea and loved me.

My new relaxed approach was finally rewarded when I succeeded in having a normal bowel movement. A nurse had anticipated this moment by warning me never to flush the toilet because, she said, "I need to look at anything you pass."

How grossly embarrassing, I had thought to myself. "Why do you have to do that?" I asked.

"I have to look at and describe any feces."

On this evening of my success, I was prepared. "Oh, let me help you," I urged the nurse. "As a creative writing instructor, I can be a big help to the hospital staff. I can teach you nurses to avoid boring, tedious patients' charts. We'll give my medical records a touch of literary merit at least. Just write, 'The brown log floated placidly past a grayish pebble in an amber pool . . .' "

We laughed together.

* * *

Time slid by, interrupted only occasionally by outside realities. One of these realities came packaged as a former high-school classmate; the word eccentric only begins to describe him. Art's shiny dome poked furtively around the door. Sneaking in to avoid the nurses, he moved like a figure in a spy movie—a sleuth running on tiptoes. He slipped sideways into the room, gliding like a late evening's shadow over the "No Visitors" sign. "I heard you were here and had to see you," he explained in a half-whisper. Sam, one of our classmates who worked weekends in physical therapy, had seen my chart and had mentioned to Art, with concern, that I was hospitalized. From his tone of voice, Art had made the assumptions. "You have cancer, don't you?" he asked bluntly.

"Yes," I admitted.

"I figured that. Your Dad had cancer, right?"

I nodded.

"I just had to see you. I knew you'd be handling it well. The thing I remember from high school is your faith. I knew that'd make a difference."

After his curiosity about my health had been satisfied, we talked about our lives since high school. Right before he left my room, he remarked, "My father has prostate cancer. He's getting pretty bad."

I realized then that he had come to comfort himself, not just me—to prove to himself that a person with faith can handle cancer. I was struck with the reality that as I lay in a hospital bed, I still represented Christ—even to people who had not seen me in over fifteen years.

*   *   *

Fear of cancer was illustrated by a visit from the pastor of the church I attended as a girl. He showed that although the Bible says, "Perfect love casts out fear," fear of cancer is not miraculously eliminated when one accepts Christian principles.

The pastor hesitantly peeked around the corner of the curtain that divided my bed from my roommate's view. The expression on his face showed he was terrified of what he would find. After all, one never knew about the emotional health of "cancer victims."

"I wanted to make sure you were decent," he stammered. "I wouldn't want some man to just barge in on my wife if she were in the hospital."

He stood shifting his weight from foot to foot, speaking a series of platitudes in his ministerial voice. "We're glad to know that you will accept God's will in this matter. . . . His grace is sufficient." He asked several standard questions about my mother and about the children. Finished with the expected dialog of hospital visits, he cleared his throat and examined each flower arrangement minutely. He stole a glance at his watch. Both of us anxiously awaited the final ritual. At last he intoned, "May I have a word of prayer with you?"

"Of course." I bowed my head in relief.

He was much better at carrying on a conversation with God than with me. Perhaps that was because he considered it acceptable to engage in a monolog with the Lord. I was sure this pastor had never considered the verse, "Be still, and know that I am God."

He finished his prayer with a dramatic crescendo—gaining confidence now that the visit was almost completed. Then he added a polishing touch. He set a copy of the devotional booklet *Daily Bread* on my bedstand, saying, "This book has three months of daily devotions. They're very uplifting. I do hope you are out of here before you use them all."

I could not cover my amusement at the implication.

"You know what I mean," he fumbled as he fled from the room.

✳   ✳   ✳

The real world impinged on my days of solitary nausea not just through occasional visitors but also through one particular televison program. Normally, as roommates or my family watched shows, I slept or lay with eyes unfocused. But one night I targeted in on the figures on the screen as contestants dressed in plunging necklines paraded on a runway. It was the Miss Universe contest. Half-jokingly, I turned to Rex. "When I get well I'm going to start a movement protesting prejudice against mastectomy patients in advertising and television programming."

He gestured in exasperation. "Sounds like another one of your ridiculous schemes. What brought that idea on?"

I explained. "Well, here I lie with an amputation I can't look at and can barely think about, and there strut dozens of women with exposed cleavage. How am I supposed to compete? If the gays can have their movement, certainly we mastectomy patients can have ours!"

Outwardly I laughed. But inwardly I cried for the young mastectomy patient who was unmarried and the older divorced or widowed woman who wanted to remarry. How could these women cope? And what of a woman whose husband valued her body over her person?

As if sensing my thoughts, Rex leaned close to assure me, "You don't have to compete for me. You already have me."

I nestled my head against his bowed forehead. "I'm grateful for that. But I'll never again be able to say that all you want me for is my body—unless you go in for bearded women."

"Can't you ever be serious?" Rex groaned.

"Not yet, honey," I admitted. "I can't be serious yet."

I was angry that the television program had intruded into my nest in room 321 and had reminded me of my deformity.

I pulled back into the cocoon of hospital routine, avoiding the prodding insistence of these occasional interruptions from the outer world. Hospital routine revolved around my two daily dressing changes. To me the biggest problem was the irritation from the surgical tape. My skin was raw even though each nurse had a new suggestion—a different kind of tape, a different position for the strips of tape, a way to use less tape while keeping the bandage secure. But to the nurses the biggest problem of the dressing changes was the fact that I never looked at my chest. Judy was the most overtly concerned that I wasn't "facing the facts" of my surgery.

I tried to clarify my reasons for avoiding seeing the graft. "You nurses have to check out your stitches to make sure the doctor did a good job. But I'm an English teacher. All I need is a verbal description."

I sensed she didn't understand, so I went on.

"My casualness about cancer doesn't mean that I don't know what's going on. And my refusal to look at my chest doesn't mean I'm denying the fact that I'm missing a breast."

"But," she insisted, "wouldn't it be better to look when you have the staff for support rather than waiting to catch a glimpse by mistake when you're alone?"

"I'm good at avoiding mirrors," I said. "My body wasn't so great before. I managed to keep my eyes off it."

"Even if you can avoid it, wouldn't you be better off looking than imagining?"

Flippantly I answered, "If I get curious in the next twenty years or so, I'll look then."

She seemed frustrated, so I tried to explain that stitches and scabs on anyone bothered me. I preferred to wait until I had a nice flat white scar like the Reach for Recovery lady.

But when Dr. Coulter told me he would discharge me on Sunday, I had misgivings about my refusal to look. I knew that unless I looked at least once the nurses would always doubt my acceptance of my surgery. They had befriended me and my family for three very critical weeks. Nurses like Bobbi and Susan had intimately molded their lives to ours. I owed them my loyalty. Looking at my chest had become a test of whether I would continue to fulfill my obligations to friendship.

I told Rex I couldn't leave without looking at least once. "Looking will be my gift to these friends."

Even though Rex disagreed, stressing that at that point in my life I was responsible for doing what was best for myself, on Sunday morning, as Judy changed the dressing for the last time, I glanced down. "I guess it's not so awful," I said. She barely contained her ecstasy.

But to myself I admitted, *perhaps Rex was right once again.*

Home
Again

LYING STILL SO AS NOT TO ROUSE MY NAUSEA, WATCHING THE
elderly woman in the bed beside me, I thought:

Today I can go home. How long has it been since I came to this
hospital room? Three weeks exactly—twenty-one days! Impossible. It seems more like a lifetime ago that I sank my toes into our
blue bedroom carpet or sat sipping tea at my own kitchen table.

Today I can relax on the sofa with Renae and Neil. Today I can
gaze at the maples guarding the perimeter of our yard. Today I
can play a Chopin melody on my piano. Today I can wear clothes
—real street clothes!

And tonight—tonight I will hear Renae mumbling in her sleep
and Neil kicking the footboard as he flops over in his bed. Tonight, when I wake, the security light will shine through the bathroom window into the hall and into my eyes. Tonight, if I lie still,
I can listen to Rex's rhythmic breathing as he lies curled on his
right side.

And tomorrow I'll listen to Rex's pickup leave for work. To-morrow I'll see the outfits the children wear to school. Tomor-row my Grandma Julian, my mother's mother, will be my private nurse.

But right now moving from this bed to the bathroom seems a monumental journey. At this moment life's ordinary activities are overwhelming.

I had nested so long in this hospital room that independence was frightening. Here I had lounged as my dressing was changed twice a day. The ringing of a buzzer brought a tea bag, a Saltine or an arm to steady my wobbling body. As much as I had fought to go home, my preparing to leave forced me to admit that there was security in the hospital's care. How could I face having to change the bandage with just Rex assisting? Genny had offered to help me, but I hated being dependent on her.

I brushed the hair from my eyes and the doubts from my mind. I would only deal with immediate problems, not think of future ones.

Mom rushed in from early church services to help me dress. She brought a loose-fitting blazer so that I could easily slip my arm into the sleeve, and slacks with an elasticized waist so that I could slide them over my abdominal incision comfortably. I attempted to slip on the bra from Reach for Recovery. Even though it was front-closing, I still needed Mom's assistance be-cause my arms were not strong enough to fasten the clasp. Al-though the front seam was padded by thick layers of cotton, the pressure still sent pain through the center incision. Mom helped me protect the area with more layers of cotton. Trying to find a way to get comfortable, I said, "Now I understand why Dr. Coulter apologized for having to cut exceptionally low. I'll bet surgeons plan incisions so that the scar is hidden under the bra line."

Wincing with pain, I surrendered at last and dressed without a bra. As I passed the mirror, I paused to see if my braless style was too apparent. I stared at my reflection. My clothes hung on me as if they were still draped over a clothes hanger. I couldn't believe it. All those days of forcing tasteless food down my throat, and I still looked like a dressed skeleton.

Judy came in to check my dressings and to give me my final instructions for home care. I was swept with a wave of nostalgia as I realized that these friends who had shared some of my most intimate moments would fade out of my life. Ignoring my emotions, I turned to ask Judy where I could weigh myself. She flew from the room and whizzed back within moments, pushing a portable scale. "Service with a smile."

"I could have walked to the storage area."

"I wanted your last memories to be those of being pampered by dedicated nurses."

I laughed. I knew I would always cherish my memories of these sensitive ones.

I stepped on the scale and adjusted the weights. I stared. I readjusted the balance. Eighteen pounds lighter. It was unbelievable! Even though I had been obsessed with eating everything that my teeth would chew, I had still lost all that weight.

"No wonder I'm weak and dizzy," I said. My voice rose. "I'm not staying a rack of bones. As long as I don't heave it back up, I'm going to gag down every bite I can shovel in."

* * *

My family breezed in. Rex had already completed the discharge forms. Our two children, Kris and my mother rushed out with luggage and flowers. Rex clasped a planter and beamed at me while Judy pushed my wheelchair.

The brightness of the outdoors blinded me as Judy wheeled my chair through the emergency room exit. The fresh autumn air filled my lungs and caressed my cheeks. A film seemed washed away from the wooded scene I had stared at each day from my window. Cotton candy clouds floated just above my grasp. The vibrant world pulsated with life, and I remained a part of it.

I felt like a princess being helped into her waiting carriage as Rex, smiling, held out his hand after opening the door of our green Duster. The prince of my dreams bowed. "Your chariot awaits you, Madam." Visions of court faded and reality impinged as my real-life prince asked, "Are you sure you're up to sitting in McDonald's? You look tired. We could go on home and ask Grandma Durney to take the children out for lunch."

I paused to consider this. It would be nice to get settled at home without the noisy confusion of children. "I am tired," I agreed. "But just in case I have to come back some day, I want the children to have good memories of my leaving the hospital. We went to McDonald's for lunch when you admitted me; we'll go now that I'm discharged."

"I hope all this fuss about the kids' attitude is unnecessary. Don't talk about going back."

Our children bounced excitedly in the back of Mom's Vega station wagon as we followed them the several blocks to the restaurant. In the parking lot, we had barely halted when Renae and Neil bounded from Mom's car, threw my passenger door open and held out their hands, fighting to escort me.

"We'll help you, Mom," Renae offered. "We're used to helping Grandma Julian."

Well, I thought, at the moment my stamina is little different from that of an eighty-year-old woman, so I guess the comparison is appropriate.

Abruptly Renae halted. "Have you looked in the mirror today, Mommy?" she asked.

"Yes, why?"

"You usually don't go anywhere with your hair looking like that."

Automatically I rearranged a couple of twiggy locks. "This is a different kind of day, honey. Are you going to be embarrassed because my hair doesn't look nice?"

"No, I just thought you might want to stay in the car if you knew what you look like."

"Well, if you aren't embarrassed, I'm going in to sit with all of you."

We shuffled slowly up the sidewalk. The smell of greasy french fries made me weave slightly as Renae held the door for me. The crowd's chatter seemed deafening after the hospital's relative solitude. I was flooded with a sense of freedom. No longer confined to a bed, a room, a floor of a building, I was free to move—

as free as my body would allow.

I sipped a milkshake and fought nausea. Soon the children were collecting the papers to throw away and arguing over who would get the front seat of Grandma's car.

On our drive home, Rex and I were accompanied only by plants and baggage. Poignant memories returned as we neared the cemetery where Dad is buried. "Let's put some of my flowers on Dad's grave," I suggested.

"I'll do it for you if you'll stay in the car." Rex drove down the winding paths and stopped in front of the headstone marked *Albert George Durney, July 26, 1920—November 26, 1967.*

Dad has left us more to remember him by than that stone, I thought. "Help me, Lord, to engrave pleasant memories on the lives around me."

Rex drove on. A comfortable stillness settled between us. I leaned back against the headrest, but I could not close my eyes. I felt like a tourist. The scenes that we passed should have been familiar. I had lived on the border of Ohio and Western Pennsylvania for thirty of my thirty-three years, leaving only when I attended college and when Rex was in the Air Force. In fact, I was born in a farmhouse about halfway between Greenville and Andover. But today all seemed foreign, as unfamiliar as if I were seeing the area for the first time.

Nearing Andover, we passed Ron and Ann's farm. I would have loved to stop and share my excitement with them. As if reading my mind, Rex said, "I talked to Ron last night and told him you were coming home. He said he would tell Ann. I wish I could have told them both in person."

"Well, at least my problems were good for something. They've given Ann and Ron something to talk about and agree upon."

Rex's eyes glistened.

When we turned onto our road, I strained to catch the first glimpse of our home. Finally I spotted our rambling white farmhouse, surrounded by maples and backed by two long loafing barns. Our home—what wealth! The marigolds swayed rhythmically in the flower bed under the yellow-curtained kitchen window. The lawn rolled like a green carpet past the two red barns neatly tucked at the back of the lot.

Basking in the tranquility of our farm, I sighed, thinking how fortunate we were to be caretakers of this fifty-two acres. "Isn't it strange how a few weeks can change a person's whole perspective?" I voiced my thoughts to Rex. "Three weeks ago I would have described our place as old and needing repairs. I would have concentrated on the mortgage payment, the lumps in the lawn, the weeds in the flower bed and the hole in the barn roof. Now all those things are unimportant beside the beauty of our home. I wonder if I'll stay so optimistic."

Rex just smiled, not answering, for perhaps there was no answer. Or perhaps neither of us wanted to admit that we would soon settle back into taking our blessings for granted.

Rex firmly gripped my arm. The three children and Mom each grabbed a bag or a plant, and we paraded up the long walk to the laundry room door. As I stepped into the kitchen, I compulsively ran my hand over the once familiar items—the stove, the refrigerator, the table. Passing the piano in the dining room, I ran my fingers over the keys.

"Play a song," Renae begged.

I sat down and began a halting rendition of "Holy, Holy, Holy." Rex beamed. I could only play simple chords, for my left arm barely pivoted at the elbow. Pain kept me from pressing firmly on the keyboard.

"I'll help you upstairs so you can rest," Rex said as I stood up.

"No, I'll just sit down here and enjoy being home."

"I'll get your robe and slippers," Neil volunteered.

"I want to stay dressed just a while longer. Thank you anyway."

I walked from the piano into our spacious living room. The oranges and yellows of the carpet smiled at me; the walls glowed. The corn field and woods in the valley seen through the ten-foot-wide bow window looked like a photograph. The plaid sofa and chair I had reupholstered four years before looked as if they belonged in a furniture showroom. The children's fingerprints on the double window over the window seat reassured me.

Snuggled under the afghan Wanda had made as a love gift several years before, I gazed at my familiar surroundings—the children's name plaques on the wall, the decoupage of Christ's hands that my sister had made for us one Christmas, the macramé owl and the large plant hanger made by friends, the copper portrait of Rex and me made in Turkey another lifetime ago and the print of a covered bridge that Mom had bought me just a few months before. Beneath the bridge was the inscription "Slow me down, Lord." I wonder if Mom realized how quickly—and through what means—that prayer would be answered, I thought.

Neil bounded past me, slid into reverse and stopped for a kiss. I knew my presence emphasized the reality of my getting better. I wanted to use my reserves to re-establish order quickly —to convince the little ones that their world was unthreatened. As if reading my mind, Rex said, "We have beans to can, kids. Come help me pick." They scampered to the garden.

While Rex, Kris and the children processed the beans, Mom drove to Greenville to pick up Grandma Julian. Since I was a little girl, Grandma has always sensed my needs. My stay in the hospital was no different. On that first evening when I called her, her gentle love crossed the telephone wires. She visited me only occasionally because she wanted me to avoid strain. When she did come, she sat quietly by my side, expecting nothing of me. On one visit, she brought me a dainty necklace, obviously carefully selected. "I wanted to get you something that will always remind you that I love you." I imagined she understood my unexpressed feelings about the flowers that died and the candy that sat untouched because of my nausea.

Although she did not talk about my illness, there was sorrow in her gray eyes. She gently touched my hair in a tender caress. "Would you like me to make you some tapioca pudding?" she offered.

"I'd love some tomorrow, Grandma—when I'm less nauseated." The lamplight cast a sheen on the waves of my grandmother's gray hair. It formed a halo on my guardian angel.

As Grandma adjusted my afghan and pillows, I sensed in her the same reaction that my father had had at the fatal car accident of Rex's sixteen-year-old sister Pam. Pam's death had been more difficult for Dad to accept than his own terminal illness. So many times Dad talked about life as a cycle, the young picking up the work that the older generation has not completed. Similarly, Grandma Julian could have faced her own illness easier than mine.

At 8:30 Rex instructed the children to take their baths and dress for bed. "We've had a busy day and tomorrow is school," he explained. When they were in pajamas, I slowly pulled myself up the stairs to tuck them in as I had always done before my hospitalization. Excited to have me home, they chattered nonstop until Rex insisted that they settle down.

I dragged myself to our room to sit on our bed for a moment. Admitting to myself that I was too weak to make another round trip to the couch, I said, "I guess I might as well stay up here, too."

"I'll turn the lights out and be right back up." Rex clomped down the stairs and quickly returned.

Rex—gardening, canning, organizing housework, tucking children in bed. Only the month before, I'd said that I knew he'd never "go domestic." How little credit I had given him. A Bible verse, "All things work together for good to them that love God," applied to our situation. I had feared Rex would be insensitive. Instead he had become my gentle protector. Cancer was drawing our family together, doing more than I ever could.

For three weeks I had looked forward to this night when I could again sleep with my husband. But our cozy romantic evening became complicated because I needed to roll to my right side to get up. To avoid waking Rex to help me if I wanted out of bed, I crawled in on "his side." But then the pillows on which I propped my arm separated us. Even though we were in the same bed, we could only touch toes.

"I feel like we're the couple in an old-fashioned 'bundling' party, all wrapped up with a board between them. With this pile of pillows, I think we're as safe from each other as they were."

"Oh, so you think you're safe," Rex growled as he raised himself over the pillows to plant a succulent kiss on my lips.

Steadily I calculated my reaction to his touch. I did not pull away. I did not wince. But the jarring of the bed sent pain through my chest. Within moments Rex drifted off to sleep, content to have me home. Shifting with insomnia, I listened to Rex's rhythmic breathing. Kris's radio played softly until after two o'clock. I smiled at the familiar night noises—the children turning in their beds, the distant barking of Spotty and Lady as they hunted in the woods behind our fields.

"Thank you for our family, Father. Is love one of the treasures we can lay up in heaven?"

"You're beginning to understand."

I dozed, but woke startled at Rex's every movement. For years we had slept sandwiched back to stomach, flipping together as one of us needed a change of position. I feared that when Rex was sound asleep he might automatically throw his arm across my shoulder and accidentally hit my incision.

On the wrong side of the bed for him, he slept fitfully. My constant change of temperature, causing me to pull a blanket up and then throw it off minutes later, also disturbed him.

Both of us alternated sleeping and waking. Periodically Rex asked, "Are you O.K., honey?"

"Mmm hmh," I'd murmur and he'd nap once more.

On Wednesday Mom took Grandma home; for even though Grandma acted pert, orchestrating the activities of a family had drained her. Then Mom drove me to my appointment with the surgeon.

I was terrified of this office visit, for I knew that the doctor planned to remove the sutures from the breast incision. I dreaded the possibility of a tender stitch. But as the nurse began snipping and pulling threads, I was aware of a wooden numbness in my chest. I felt inanimate.

The nurse, removing alternate stitches from the graft site, worked up to the underarm area. "Move your arm away from your body so that I can reach these sutures," she ordered as she attempted to swivel my arm out. I cringed in pain.

"Stop! I'll do it."

With my right hand, I tried to inch my arm out from my body. Watching me, the nurse swirled and called down the hall, "Doctor, come back here quickly, please."

He ambled back into the examining room.

"Doctor," the nurse dramatically announced, "this woman has a frozen shoulder."

I panicked. I wasn't wooden any longer. Now I was a block of ice. She pronounced her ominous words in a disgusted tone, but the doctor remained unshocked.

"Let me show you a couple of exercises to do," he said, demonstrating. "Let your arm swing like a pendulum in larger and larger circles each day. Then hold your hand on the center of your chest, lean over and swing your elbow in larger and larger circles. Do you understand?"

I nodded dumbly, grateful for his calmness.

"Do the exercises in the Reach for Recovery booklet too. That will keep you busy until you come back for your next visit."

The doctor sidled out.

"You are much too young to lose the use of your arm," the nurse resumed. "I've seen women who didn't exercise enough become permanently crippled. I'd hate to see that happen to you."

She lectured on as I dressed, telling me to brush my hair several times a day with my left hand. My arm would benefit and so would my hair. She scolded me in a pseudosweet voice and ended by shaking her head woefully and saying, "Tsk, tsk." She was the ruling despot in her sphere, and her tone simultaneously humiliated and angered me.

I showed no emotion as the nurse solicitously guided me to the receptionist to schedule my next appointment. Icily I finished the necessary clerical work. I was settled in the front seat of Mom's car before I began to sob. Mom, surprised, said nothing. She waited patiently for me to explain.

"I tried so hard."

"I'm sure you did, honey. What's wrong?"

"The nurse said I have a frozen shoulder. Why didn't the doctor start me on exercises earlier? I didn't know I was stiffening up. Now it'll be twice as hard to exercise. What if I'm too late? What if I'm crippled like the nurse said I might be?"

Mom listened quietly for several minutes, knowing I expected no answers.

"I'm sure you'll be fine. It may take hard work, but you've

never been afraid of work," she encouraged me.

I sniffled.

"We'll stop at the Dairy Queen for lunch, O.K.?"

"I don't want anything." I whined like a spoiled child.

"You can sit in the car. I'll go in and get anything you want."

After a few more minutes of pouting, I ordered a hot fudge sundae. I picked at it, stirring the ice cream into swirled designs. On the way home, I alternated between complaining, staring straight ahead, pretending I was napping and, occasionally, attempting civility. I knew I was making it difficult for Mom, but I was too busy being upset about my "frozen shoulder" to care. And I knew mother loved me even when I did act like a baby.

Rex's pickup followed Mom's station wagon into our driveway. He had rushed home for lunch to hear what the doctor had said at my appointment. I told him that the nurse had scolded me for having a stiff shoulder. "The Reach for Recovery lady said to wait until the doctor ordered the exercises, but he never did."

Rex's voice began to rise. "The doctor shouldn't have had to tell you to begin exercising in moderation. You're an adult."

I snapped back, "Start yelling. Of course, resort to the typical Britton method of handling a problem. Don't you think I'm upset enough without your criticism?"

"But I told you to start exercising, and now you act shocked that someone else tells you the same thing."

"The old 'I told you so' routine. You always know what I should do. I have to be perfect. I'm supposed to be superwoman. But you're as healthy as a horse, and you can't get up off the couch to change your own TV channels."

Rex glared at me as when disciplining one of our children. "Who's yelling now? Grow up!"

"I should have known your understanding wouldn't last. I should have known you'd go back to your old ways of handling problems. I wanted your support—not your criticism. No matter what you say, I'm not going to apologize for being sick. I won't tolerate your hassle anymore."

Rex did not know how to handle my unexpected attack. "I

don't have to stay here and listen to this," he said. "I can go back to work."

This was where I always gave in. But this time I remained stubborn. "Then go. I'm not begging you to stay."

Rex hesitated a moment and I glowered at him. Then he swiveled on his heels and stomped to the door, slamming it hard enough to rattle the vase sitting on the kitchen windowsill. I stood panting in anger and exhaustion. The pickup roared as he revved the engine. Gravel flew as he shifted into reverse.

I turned away from my mother. We had never argued so openly in front of her.

Within minutes, Rex's pickup coughed back into the driveway. He slammed the door as he re-entered and stood, jaw rigid and hands on hips, waiting for me to say something. I was silent.

"Now are you ready to talk sensibly?" he began.

"If you don't like what I have to say, then leave again," I answered evenly.

He shook his head, obviously not understanding me, and pulled up a chair beside me. "Would you fix a sandwich for me?" he asked Mom.

Turning back to me, he reached for my hand. I melted. "I'm so scared and tired. And then I get yelled at like a lazy child."

After Rex left for work, I apologized to Mom for subjecting her to such a scene. "But I can't have him treating me like an invalid or worse yet like a child that he can scold. I'm his wife. I will not be patronized." I propped one elbow on the table and stared at my reflection in the toaster. My tantrums had exhausted me.

Genny arrived to change my dressing. I narrated the nurse's tirade and asked why Dr. Coulter hadn't started my exercises in the hospital. Defending the doctor, Genny said that opinions vary on when to start the exercise program. Often the area becomes swollen and inflamed from too strenuous exercise too early, causing delay of full use of the arm. Then she began to instruct me, demonstrating variations of the doctor's swivel exercises and adding advice on walking the wall with my fingertips and pulling a rope over the top of a door. I gritted my teeth and awkwardly imitated her.

Genny stopped and warned me. "Don't exercise past the point of discomfort. Just be consistent and sensible and you'll do better."

"But the nurse said the shoulder is frozen. I could be permanently impaired."

"Now, Janet, just relax. You know that anything that freezes can thaw." She hugged me, and I was reassured by her touch. Of course she was right. That's why the doctor didn't appear disturbed.

Exhausted, I propped up my arm and sunk back into thought. Engulfed in nausea, barely able to climb the stairs to my bedroom or read a book or enjoy a phone conversation—and I must exercise!

I reached for the soft sponge-rubber ball that I squeezed to strengthen my arm. It was in sad shape. Spotty had chewed a hole in it when trying to wrestle it away from Neil. When I tired of squeezing it, I used my right hand to prop my left arm farther away from my side. I determined to stretch it out a little more each day, staying right at the threshold of pain until I could extend my left arm straight over my head. I could use my resting time to exercise. I began to believe I'd make it. Mentally I relaxed.

My frozen shoulder would thaw.

* * *

The next morning I lay in bed inching my arm away from my body and contemplating the strange fact that several close friends had not stopped by yet. I regretted not having informed all these friends about the events of my hospitalization. I vowed to dial at least three before I took a nap—Terri, Kathleen and Nancy. I kept the conversations short because I tired quickly and my purpose was simply to show that I valued each of them.

Within five minutes after hanging up the phone, I heard Nancy's "Woohoo" at the door. She had dashed right over to see me. She said that previously she had stayed away because of the stories she had heard about my emotional condition. "What people were saying didn't sound like the Janet I know. But cancer is such a trauma. It would have been understandable if you had reacted differently than I expected."

Nancy outlined the reasoning of the grapevine. First, I had sneaked away without publicizing the nature of my surgery, although a compilation of all of the facts pointed to cancer. Then one avid reader analyzed my actions according to Dr. Kübler-Ross's theory in *Death and Dying*. All my behavior, the grapevine surmised, fit the typical responses of the terminally ill: (1) shock and denial, (2) anger, (3) bargaining, (4) depression (according to this group, I had not yet reached stage 5, acceptance). For example, the "No Visitors" rule was interpreted three ways. Some said I was denying my illness and refusing to discuss my cancer. Others said I was exhibiting anger and avoiding people so as not to lash out at them. A third group saw the rule as a cover for my deep depression and withdrawal from society. Their application of Kübler-Ross's book led them to request that others "pray for Janet's acceptance."

I decided that the best way to handle the rumors was to let people see me personally. The sooner I was into a normal routine, the sooner the stories would end. So Saturday morning I announced, "I'm going to ask Gail to do my hair. I'm going to church. I can sit for an hour in a pew just as well as I can sit on our sofa."

As Gail styled my hair, she succinctly summarized the coffee-shop gossip. "You know—what a shame it is for a young woman like you with two darling children to only have months to live." The circles under my eyes the Sunday morning before I went to the hospital were proof of my terminal condition.

"But I've looked that way a thousand times before," I protested.

"But you've never been a cancer victim before."

Yes, that one fact does change people's perceptions of an individual.

That evening while Mom supervised the children's baths, I propped myself in the recliner to finish reading the literature distributed by Reach for Recovery. One section struck me:

Yours is a hidden scar. If you REACH to help yourself, if you understand and truly believe that you *can,* no one need know that you have had a mastectomy unless you choose to tell them. And those who do know—your husband, children, people you love—they will have a chance to love you even more because you are so special to them.

I knew what the pamphlet had intended to stress. How much more fortunate to be like me rather than like one of my fellow teachers who stepped on a land mine in Vietnam. He is labeled by his double amputations even by strangers. I had a hidden amputation of a body part. But I found the literature's emphasis ironic. Privacy was certainly a good theory, unless a person lived in a small town. Here what information you don't know, you just ad lib as you go along.

In bed that night I started to repeat the gossip I had heard about. Rex stopped me. "Forget the rumors. All that matters is that you're home with the children and me. Forget other people."

Of course he was right. I concentrated on seducing my husband. I needed to feel whole again. I wanted him to handle me like a woman, not a delicate piece of crystal. I clung to him, once again a wife. Contentedly, I purred.

"You need your sleep for tomorrow," Rex murmured.

I agreed, but I couldn't sleep. I was home. I was surrounded by people who loved me. I had the husband millions of women search for. Yet I could not shake my anger at being emotionally dissected by people I didn't even know.

"Lord, you have given me everything, but I'm losing my peace."

"Your mind must be stayed on me."

I hummed "Great Is Thy Faithfulness." I repeated my verse, "Whatsoever things are good..." When my concentration slipped even momentarily, I was smothered by coffee-shop rumors.

I attempted to escape undetected to the bathroom. Carefully I inched my feet to the edge of the bed. I lowered my right foot onto the floor. I pulled my right arm under me and inched my body up. I slid my left foot toward the floor.

"What's the matter?" Rex catapulted upright. "Where are you going?"

"To the bathroom, honey. Go back to sleep."

I drank a glass of water and checked our sleeping children. Returning, I slowly lowered my body onto the bed, trying not to wake Rex or my pain. I readjusted myself, propping my pillows to give me the greatest comfort. But once again my mind went out of control, careening to the gossip.

Was I fooling myself about my motives for privacy? Did I really want to spare my family from the torture I had gone through with Dad's illness, or was I simply sensitive to everyone's knowing of my missing breast?

All the emotions I had been suppressing rushed to the surface. In the hospital I had flippantly told Harry to use the Mark Twain quote, "the rumors of my death have been greatly exaggerated," to report my condition in Sunday's announcements. Now the humor of the situation eluded me. I felt pinned to the wall, my every move scrutinized. If I was cheerful, I would be viewed as not accepting the reality of my imminent death. If I was tired or depressed, it would be evidence that my mental health was eroding; I would be criticized for "not holding up for the family."

But in spite of my anger, I had to accept the fact that I had lost my battle for privacy. Since I refused to be a hermit, I had no choice but to deal with everyone else's hang-ups as well as my own. So—I had to be on stage. I must not look tired, I thought. I must not be angry or depressed. I must remember that every bout of the common cold will result in rumors that I'm having a recurrence of cancer. If I go into public angry at Rex for not taking out the garbage, my cloudy expression will be interpreted as depression over cancer. Those were the facts. I must hide behind a stone mask.

"Child, you are torturing yourself."

"I can't help it, Father."

"Let me help it, child."

I dozed.

*   *   *

I dressed for church as carefully as I had for my Junior Prom. From the assortment of blousy tops and dresses that Mom had collected for me to wear, I chose a rose-pink outfit with a high neckline and a fully gathered top. In it I felt comfortably hidden from curious scrutiny.

Kris and I took the lamb's wool from the pocket of the Reach for Recovery bra and began the task of stuffing the left side of a feminine front-closing padded bra that Genny had bought for me.

"I think it needs a little more on the inside," Kris suggested as she stood back to check the symmetry of my bosom.

Laughing, I said to her, "Of course you'd be better at this than me. You're more artistic!"

A friendly murmur spread through the congregation as my family guided me into the sanctuary during the singing of the first hymn. As I settled into the pew, my strength dissipated. I read the words to the hymns but could not sing. I consciously used both hands equally as I alternated pulling a sweater around my shoulders with fanning myself with a bulletin. Hot and cold and hot and cold, I could not concentrate on worship. Rex leaned over and whispered, "Your left side is higher." Discreetly, I wiggled the bra into place.

After the benediction, friends swarmed around me, welcoming me back. The children glowed.

Exhausted, I smiled placidly as a casual acquaintance said, "It took my sister-in-law several months to recover when she had the operation you did."

My guard slipped. A surge of curiosity penetrated my defenses and I prodded. "Oh, really? What surgery are you referring to?"

"Why, your hysterectomy, of course," she answered and continued relaying the saga of her sister-in-law's misery.

The situation struck me as ludicrous. Details had certainly been confused in the maze of misinformation. But a uterus or an ovary or a breast—all female organs were lumped together in most people's minds. Even if I had called a town meeting and given a lecture on my surgeries, including charts and illustrations, people would still have improvised the facts.

Abruptly Sally interrupted. "What was all the secrecy about your hospital stay?" she demanded. "When you're in the hospital that long, cancer is just logical." She insisted that my friends had the right to know all the details of my illness.

I told her that I felt my friends should respect my desire for privacy. Respect for the other person's wishes is essential to true friendship.

Sally thought I was wrong. When she had had an accident, she said, she needed to tell her friends all the details so that they could pray.

"But the Great Physician knows all the facts of the case already," I said. "I'm sure simply praying for my recovery is effective. No one has to tell God what needs healing." I would not back down.

Reluctantly she agreed, but quickly added that in addition to the need for prayers was the need to talk about the problem. After her accident, Sally had found even a stranger's concern comforting.

"Then for Sally it's important to discuss the details of illness," I responded. "But I'm Janet. I need to talk about my children, about the weather, about everyday trivia. We're different."

I couldn't help comparing Sally's remarks to those of the sloppy nurse who had changed my first dressing. That nurse did not understand that while some people should cry, others, like me, should joke. Like that nurse, some of my friends were telling me what I should feel and what I should want, trying to fit me into the stereotype of a "cancer victim." I tried to explain to Sally that just as parents know that each of their children needs different treatment (one needs a swat on the bottom and another needs to sit quietly in a chair), so also friends need to be sensitive to each other's unique personality.

Other well-wishers interrupted Sally's and my conversation. "God has to heal you. I just couldn't believe in his goodness if he didn't." "I just don't understand why a sweet lady like you should get sick." "I'm going to pray for your faith so that you'll be healed." Surely just as people were trying to squeeze my personality into a box, so they were also trying to force God to conform to their perception of him. Prayers were obviously being hurled at God like commands. Surely God *will* heal you! (The unstated additions were either *if* you have faith or *if* he has power.) My spirits sank further.

Rex whisked me home and settled me, like an invalid, in our recliner. I feared I would suffocate under the cloud of confusion brought on by all the comments. I would have liked to say, as Job did to his friends, "Miserable comforters are you all." In the name of comfort and concern, friends clustered about gossiping, digging for details, analyzing my psyche and making judgmental innuendos about my emotional and spiritual condition. In the same way, they subtly attacked God.

Many were ignoring the fact that illness and death were never intended for God's creation. Originally God shaped a perfect world for us. But he also created us with free will, and we chose sin and death. The suffering in this world is the product of the Fall. God doesn't deliberately send us the pain. But he does use the grief of an imperfect world to draw us to him—to remind us that all is unimportant compared to the development of our love for him and for other people. The imperfect world will pass away, but God and his people will live forever. Out of the world's evil God works good in our personal lives. Although God never intended the suffering, he uses it to strengthen our inner selves.

God teaches us like the mother eagle teaches her young. As the eaglet grows, the mother eagle begins throwing out the cushioning feathers and grass so that the sticks prick and make the babies less complacent. Eventually the little birds squirm about and try their wings. When they fail in their early attempts, the mother swoops under them and bears them back to the nest until another day when they are stronger and try again, this time successfully.

Dad's death furnished early opportunities for me to test my wings. And when I failed, God swooped down, soothed my pain and fear, and picked me up until I grew stronger.

Viewing my life, I saw that my Father had been carefully preparing me to deal with my own illness. Like a good parent, little by little he allowed the pricking world to force me to try my wings again and again. Many times after Dad's death I had been in danger of dashing my brains out on the rocks below my nest.

For example, while Rex guarded the perimeters of the Air

Force base with his police dog, I lay in our Turkish basement apartment and demanded that God heal Dad who was suffering in the last stages of cancer. I quoted Christ's own words to him: "If you ask me anything in my name, I will do it." At times I argued logically, "How can Dad reach others for you if he is dead?" Other times logic dissolved into emotion. I cried; I begged; I insisted. "Please let Dad live to be the grandfather to our children. Please let our family enjoy his sense of humor just a while longer. Please, please, please. . . ."

Then one late November afternoon, just four months after our marriage, Rex returned from the base with a telegram in his hand. Dad had died three days before.

Wings flapping wildly, I plummeted under the weight of guilt; I had failed in my intercession. Mentally I flagellated myself with the biblical phrase, "Oh ye of little faith." Then momentarily the knowledge of God's character would buoy me up. How could God, the God of love, condemn my father to death because of his daughter's inadequacies? I couldn't be responsible.

My upward flutter was transient. I dipped at the thought, "But if I haven't failed, then God has. Perhaps he's impotent—no more effective than a stone or wooden idol."

As I skimmed the rocks below me, a letter from Mom, telling of a powerful God answering my parents' prayers, swooped under me.

For weeks Mom had spent every moment in the hospital that she was not working in the store. In spite of Dad's urgings, she would not go home to sleep. The Christmas season, when the stores in Greenville would stay open twelve hours a day, six days a week, was approaching. Dad motioned his friends to his side and whispered, "Please pray that the Lord would either heal me or allow me to die by the week after Thanksgiving when Shirley has to work from nine to nine. She must have rest."

Dad died peacefully the Sunday morning after Thanksgiving. "Evidently the mass around his heart enlarged faster than I thought it would," his doctor remarked. But Mother saw an answer to prayer—both Dad's request to save her further exhaustion and her own prayer to spare Dad's suffering. For Dad, there was no final rending agony, just release from the painful prison of his body.

Mom's letter undergirded my slipping faith in God's ability to answer prayer. But I began tumbling again when I considered that, while caring for my parents' specific concerns, God had ignored me. God could have granted all our petitions simply by healing Dad by Thanksgiving. I was angry. Although outwardly I obeyed God's direct commands, I protected myself from intimate involvement with this superior Dictator who had stonily allowed my loneliness and my grief.

Then one night as I flipped through my Bible out of habit, that tiny verse, the shortest in the Bible, leaped out at me: "Jesus wept." "Why did Jesus cry?" I wondered. Certainly he knew that Lazarus was better off residing in a land with no suffering. He couldn't even have been temporarily lonely for his friend, because he knew that within moments he would resurrect Lazarus. Jesus' tears could not logically have been for Lazarus. His tears must have been for the grief of Mary and Martha, his friends. It impressed me that Jesus did not upbraid Lazarus's sisters for their lack of faith or for their selfishness in preferring to have Lazarus with them in this imperfect world. Jesus understood their pain. And he cared.

After months of harboring anger and isolation, I allowed the powerful and loving One to share my sorrow over Dad's death. Christ gave me the strength to soar above the crags. Previously when people approached me with the statement, "I was sorry to hear about your father's passing," I had always wanted to scream, "How can you be sorry? You don't have any idea what I'm going through. I miss my father's corny jokes. I miss the fact that my children will never have their grandfather to spoil them. I miss hearing his cough in church. I miss . . . Oh, you wouldn't understand." Now, at last, I acknowledged One who did understand everything. And who cared deeply. After listening to my wailing complaints, he simply held me and wept with me. God offered the greatest comfort available—the honest sharing of my grief.

Yet from these heights, I again began to falter. God suffers when I suffer. So why does he say no if it hurts him to see me sorrowful?

Years later motherhood exercised my weak wings. One day as I forced myself not to help as Neil struggled to tie a bow on his tennis shoe, I began to understand how One who loves and has the power to grant the request can still say no. Triumphantly Neil pulled a limp loop in his shoestring. Thrilled, he flung himself into my arms. "I tied my own shoe. See, Mommy, I'm a big boy now."

I celebrated with him.

Later that afternoon when I told him it was time for his nap, he stared at me with wide, innocent eyes and declared, "Big boys don't take naps. I'm a big boy now. I tie shoes."

Firmly I told him that he had to be even bigger before he could go without his nap, and I gently guided him up the stairs.

"Meany!" he screamed as I closed the door of his room. Between sobs he cried out, "You don't love me or you wouldn't make me go to bed!"

At that moment, in Neil's voice, I heard my own whining. How many hundreds of times during my father's illness and after his death had I asked, "Why, why, why? Don't you know that I want . . ." Hadn't I, in a more subtle way, been calling my heavenly Father a meany for not always giving me what I asked for? When my Father, who had promised me every "good and perfect gift," stood by while I wailed my complaints, certainly he was acting in love just as I was when I put Neil to bed for a nap, even though he didn't understand his own need for rest.

As a parent, I know how to give my children what is best for them. Renae, bolting into the house from the school bus, yells, "Mom, I'm starved. I can't wait until Dad comes home. Could I have a piece of pie now?" Although I say no to the pie, I add, "But there's fruit in the refrigerator that you can have." And slowly I realized that God, too, answers our requests in a more perfect way. Dad had asked if he could be healed, if he could have the appealing piece of pie on the counter. And his Father answered, "No, you may not have the pie now. But you are hungry; you do have a legitimate concern about Shirley. You may have the fruit which is good for you and your wife. I will bring you home with me the Sunday after Thanksgiving."

My faith strengthened, too, as I realized that sometimes a parent must say no to one child because there is something better for the whole family. We said no to an expensive race-set for Neil because the money was needed for the family's vacation to Virginia. I began to see the analogy. Dad and our immediate family wanted Dad to be healthy for many more years. But God used the illness for the family of humanity. Our purpose on this earth is to serve other people—to aid them, to comfort them and to introduce them to our heavenly Father. Dad's illness and death allowed him to reach more people in a few months than he might have reached in twenty years on the farm. People who would not attend church or open a Bible saw in Dad's life that Christ can give peace in all circumstances. I began to understand God as a parent, not deliberately causing pain, but allowing temporary discomfort for a greater good.

But in spite of the wing exercise I got in the years that I flailed about trying to understand why God permitted Dad's death, I still found my strength limited. Dealing with breast cancer, attempting to fly in an atmosphere of gossip which hurt me and distorted God's character, trying to cope with my own physical and emotional stress, I began to waver. But my Father soared to my rescue and placed me with my burdens on the back of a friend who willingly bore me: Genny, who glided in to do my daily dressing change.

"Oh, Genny, I thought I had learned to trust God's strength and love. But I get obsessed with fears and anger over unimportant things. People talk about their concern for me, and make me miserable. They pray to a God whose personality I barely recognize as that of my Father in the Bible. I get so confused."

Living by the verse, "Let us not love with words or tongue but with actions and in truth," Genny guided me back to rest on the principles I thought I had learned. She reminded me that my hormonal imbalance and weakness from surgery made me more vulnerable to stress. As she made me physically comfortable, I was lifted by her unconditional love. Genny made true friendship appear so simple.

I was saved once again from a fall. I had been tempted by others' views to see physical healing as my children see ice cream —an urgent need. I was lifted once more to understand that while physical health delights in the pleasures that last for a time, spiritual health finds joy in truths that are eternal. I was lifted to trust that God, as always, had a logical answer to each of my questions even if I didn't have the maturity to grasp his reasoning. Bombarded with questions, I remembered that "now we see through a glass, darkly. Then face to face. Now we know in part. Then in whole." I perceived that my views on God's character, on his will for my life and on death are not complete. My vision is improving, but I still know only in part.

Strengthened by years of struggle, my wings once more supported me in the winds of my own cancer. I remembered how difficult it was for Renae and Neil to learn to walk, how hard they struggled to pull themselves to a stool or to stagger between the coffee table and the sofa. And now I am constantly yelling at them to stop running in the house. What was a struggle is now taken for granted. The lessons that I fought to learn from the Bible now seem so obvious. Perhaps the struggle of learning to walk and the struggle to understand Christ's teachings are similar. And perhaps the whole concept of death is just as simple. Maybe I'll never in this world have the maturity to understand death, but some day these insurmountable questions may seem very elementary. Maybe...

* * *

Life at home settled into a pattern. I became accustomed to moving carefully to avoid dizziness, eating conservatively to lessen nausea, sleeping with my arm propped to alleviate pain, exercising to build strength. Genny nursed me. Mom organized Wednesday afternoons and Sundays. Rex supervised the household. Friends dropped in. We'd sit, talk, laugh. They'd leave. I'd collapse.

I knew I had to break out of this useless role. Anxiously I

anticipated the day I could return to the normal routine of teaching school. All of the family saw my lying in bed as an ominous sign. Kris was doing poorly in her classwork. She talked about dropping out, arguing that she hated going to school when I was home. "I wish I could stay with you. I still worry about you."

The two little ones were less obvious about their concern than Kris, but they asked questions—"Are you in bed again?" and "Aren't you going back to work?" "Substitutes are boring, Mom," they hinted.

Although Rex warned me to be cautious—"I know how you love to teach. But don't go back until you're strong"—his tense expression when he thought I wasn't watching revealed his concern. My return to normal routine would reassure him, just as it would our children.

By the fourth week of school, I was chomping at the bit. The sub visited me to discuss my classes. She was totally ignoring my carefully constructed unit plans. I felt I must return to my job as soon as possible.

"Father, am I foolish for being impatient?"

God leaned over and whispered, "Child, my Word instructs that 'Our people must learn to devote themselves to doing what is good . . . and not live unproductive lives.' You are one of my people, aren't you, Janet?"

"Of course, Father."

"You are living. You must be productive. Cancer doesn't change that command."

I was grateful for his answer. "I'm certainly ready, Father." The day of the sub's visit, I determined to return to school within two weeks. I called one of my professors at Youngstown State University, Gratia Murphy, and asked if she would give her usual yearly lecture to my classes during the week of October 16.

But my appointments for radiation therapy had to be scheduled before the doctor would allow me to go back to work. And the graft had to be healed before radiation could be scheduled. Yet in spite of my impatience for complete healing, I did not daily check my progress. I avoided glancing at the thin layer of bluish membrane that covered my chest—the graft site that looked like a baby's soft spot as my heart's pulsation rhythmically vibrated the onionskin covering. I detested my mutilation, my concave left side with the apparently bottomless canyon that had once been my armpit. I habitually waited to toss my clothes onto the floor until I was shielded from view by the shower curtain. I dried cautiously, always keeping a towel draped over my left shoulder until I had slipped my bra neatly into place. I learned to dress without exposing my former left breast as expertly as a woman nursing a child without allowing an immodest glimpse. Safe from scrutiny, the graft steadily mended.

*   *   *

Only a few scabs clung to the edges of the graft the day I picked up my records from Dr. Coulter's office to hand-carry to the radiation therapist. At home, aided by Genny's medical dictionary, I perused the documents labeled "Metastatic carcinoma left breast to axilla node." The cold facts of my case stared back through impassionate lidless eyes. When I finished, I wished I could flip to a final chapter and read the resolution of my case; I wondered where on the chart of survival rates my case would be recorded.

Impatiently I resealed the manila folder of records. I looked forward to radiation therapy, for it meant that I was that much closer to completing the medical protocol. Moving from the surgeon to the radiation therapist was a type of graduation, a move toward recovery. I was anxious to go on living, undisturbed by frequent doctor appointments. Spending so much time protecting my life, I had little time left over for living.

Rays
of
Hope

NANCY TOOK ME TO MY FIRST APPOINTMENT WITH THE RADIA-
tion therapist. I registered with the receptionist and then sat
squirming, waiting to hear my name announced. Nancy sat tranquilly knitting a sweater for a Christmas present. I barely glanced
at the room or the people around me. Eventually a matronly
nurse called my name. I followed her to an examination room.
She handed me a gown and said that the doctor would be with me
soon. I stepped into the bathroom, hung my blouse and bra on
the hook, removed the gauze bandage which comfortably con-
cealed my deformed side, and slipped the gown on. I shivered.
The moments crawled by as I waited to be sentenced. A dark,
petite woman entered. "Hello, Mrs. Britton. I'm Dr. Nath." She
wheeled her stool on its casters until she faced me, our knees
touching. I tried to determine what nationality she was—Syrian
perhaps or Pakistani. Her face was inscrutable.

"Tell me what has happened," she purred. I strained to understand her words through the unfamiliar accent.

"You mean why am I here?" I asked, unsure of her question.

"Yes, what has been your problem?" she said, a little louder.

"I brought records from my surgeon. I gave them to the receptionist."

"I know that. I want you to tell me yourself. I will read the records later."

I must have looked puzzled, for after pausing she continued. "I have found that the patient is the best source of information. Sometimes you can give the clue that has been previously overlooked by the doctors."

I understood her purpose. I began my story. "This spring I found a lump in my left breast."

"What month?"

"March, I guess."

"Where exactly was the lump? Show me," she said as she slipped the gown from my shoulders. I pointed to the lower center of where my breast had been.

"How did you find it?" she asked. "Do you do regular self-examination?"

I told her the story of the elusive chocolate-chip cookie crumb. I was extremely self-conscious about sitting naked to the waist talking to a stranger, but she reacted not at all.

After I had covered every detail of my medical history, she examined me thoroughly. Her only comment was, "This is a very neat job." At that moment I understood Dr. Coulter's careful burning of the thick growths from the edges of the skin graft. It was important to his professional reputation to keep my scars hidden and smooth.

As suddenly as the doctor had arrived, she stood and glided back out the door.

"You may get dressed," the nurse said. "The doctor will be back after she has read your records. Do you have a member of your family with you today?"

"I have a friend who's like a sister."

"Would you like her here when the doctor talks to you? Sometimes it helps if someone is with you to remember the doctor's comments."

"Well, I guess so. That'd be fine."

By the time I had finished dressing, Nancy was sitting in a chair in the examining room, still knitting. We talked until the doctor returned with her decree.

"I agree with your surgeon that you are a candidate for radiation therapy. The position of the lump is most significant. If cancer cells traveled 180 degrees to affect these lymph nodes," she pointed under my arm, "then it is only logical to assume that cancer cells also moved directly to the internal mammary chain—the lymph nodes directly beneath the sternum—because these nodes are so close to the original tumor. The internal nodes can't be felt nor can they be detected by x rays. They cannot be removed surgically so we will radiate this area. We will also radiate this area," she pointed along my shoulder, "in case lymph nodes there have been affected."

I considered her reasoning. Well, she must be right. Her diagnosis was logical. If the lump was so little but metastasis had already taken place, if the cells had traveled that distance, then they had probably traveled in other directions too.

"I want you to have a liver scan before your first treatment." She wrote on my chart as she talked. "I am scheduling you for the twenty-five-day protocol."

I couldn't believe what she was saying—twenty-five days of radiation. "Can I work?" was the first question I blurted out. "I was planning to go back to work next week."

"Sometimes a patient works part of a day. The technicians work Monday through Friday from 8:00 to 3:00. You can discuss the time with them next Monday on your first visit." School hours are 8:00 to 3:30, I thought. There was no way I could work a full day. But I'd think of some way to return to school as I'd planned. I just had to.

The doctor then explained that a major side effect of radiation is tiredness. Rapidly she listed other side effects and whipped out a small pamphlet that discussed the purposes and results of radiation therapy.

Normally full of questions, I could think of nothing to say. This was much more serious than I had anticipated.

As she finished her short lecture, she added, "Our staff believes strongly that you are a candidate for chemotherapy. Radiation will destroy cancer cells in the areas radiated. Chemotherapy is needed to destroy any cells that have traveled to other body areas."

I must have shown my shock. My thick, dry tongue would not form the questions that attacked my mind. She continued, soothingly, "This is just a prophylactic therapy—to prevent the recurrence of the disease."

* * *

I left the office weighed down by the information. "They act serious about the whole thing," I moaned to Nancy as we drove home. "Surgery, radiation, chemo, liver scans, chest x rays—a person could believe she's really sick!"

I could not fathom what lay ahead, beginning with five weeks of traveling eighty miles a day for a few minutes' treatment which would leave me weak and lethargic. But I had no choice. The doctor's statement wasn't "*if* the cancer has moved into the central nodes," but "we must destroy the cancer cells that *have spread* to the central nodes." And then I must undergo chemo? Well, someone would have to do some fast talking before I would agree to that.

As soon as Nancy left me at home, I lay across my bed and dialed the superintendent of my school district to consult him about my dilemma. "I had no idea when I planned my return that treatment would last five weeks. And I must get back to work." Then I outlined the plan that I had devised on the ride back to Andover. My afternoon schedule was the lightest of my teaching career. Ninth period was my conference period, a time for planning, grading papers and so on. Tenth period was an independent reading class. I was sure colleagues would monitor my last-period class so I could go to my treatments. If this plan to return on a full-time basis was unacceptable, I would be forced to return on half-day sick leave until I'd completed radiation.

When I had finished describing my options, the superintendent remained noncommittal, pointing out that the dean had to make the scheduling decisions in his building.

At 2:30 the next day, with dread, I approached the dean's office. He was a new administrator, and I didn't want our first meeting to focus on my cancer. Part of me felt as if I were going for an interview for my own position and another part as if I were attending my own trial—a trial to determine my value as a professional. After the initial amenities were over, I presented my case. I stressed my determination to return to a normal lifestyle, to a job I love. As I listed the advantages of using my experience for the whole day, Dean Soleman sat stonefaced, more inscrutable than the radiation therapist I had encountered the day before.

I concluded that even though I preferred to teach as much of my schedule as possible, I would go on a half-day schedule if he was concerned about my plan to leave the building early.

But if a colleague could help me cover the whole day's schedule, I'd sign up for the last radiation appointment of the afternoon. I added that I didn't expect his answer that day, but that I would need to know soon in order to schedule my treatments.

Sphinxlike, Dean Soleman stared through me. I tried to refrain from making snap judgments about this man. I wanted to be tolerant, for I knew that many people initially are uncomfortable dealing with issues involving cancer.

Abruptly he dismissed me by standing and saying, "I will get back to you tomorrow."

"Fine," I said. "I'll wait for your call." Then nervously I repeated, "You *will* call me, and I won't need to bother you."

But Wednesday and Thursday passed and the dean did not call. Thursday evening his secretary phoned to ask if I wanted my paycheck mailed or delivered by a coworker. I mentioned that Mr. Soleman had not called as he said he would. She assured me that he probably just assumed I would know that covering one period was no problem. But I stressed that I'd be more comfortable if she double-checked. "I have to set up my appointments for radiation on Monday," I said, "and my choice of appointment time depends on my teaching schedule."

"You know what a family we are around here," the secretary insisted. "We're just going to be thrilled to have you back with us. Besides, everyone knows even an excellent sub can't begin to replace an experienced master teacher."

I thanked her for her vote of confidence, pushed school from my mind and concentrated on preparing myself for the therapy that was ahead of me. I dreaded my first radiation treatment.

* * *

Monday morning at eight o'clock, Genny and I walked into the nuclear medicine department for my scheduled liver-spleen scan. Immediately after registering, I was directed to a treatment room. As the technician pressed a swab of cotton against the spot where she had injected the radioactive isotopes, I asked her, "Where should I go to take off my clothes?"

"The liver scan is done through your clothing since the machine detects only radioactivity."

I relaxed. This sounds easy, I thought.

After twenty minutes, a second technician arrived. He was one of the frozen ones—unsmiling, unresponsive. The scan was simple and painless. I lay silently on the table.

* * *

Next, Genny and I wound our way to the basement, to the radiation department. Even though the room was packed with bodies, it was as silent as a church service. Physical closeness contrasted sharply with emotional isolation. People stared straight ahead. Their blank expressions reminded me of T. S. Eliot's "Hollow Men." No humanity appeared to inhabit these empty shells.

Bizarre markings added a science-fiction air to the scene. Black X's and angles decorated the shells. The markings varied. One woman had a single X right between the eyes, as if her forehead were a target. One, with several X's marked across the jawbone, appeared to have a choppy Dutch-boy haircut. Looking at other patients, I realized that radiation in the region of the head caused the hair to break off and so determined hair style.

Some patients clung weakly to an escort's arm. Some slumped in wheelchairs. The patients were easily distinguishable from the drivers even without visible X's. A distinctive pallor and lack of agility marked the patients. But most of all their eyes—their radiation stare—marked them.

I vowed to avoid being defeated by weakness or fatigue. I vowed to walk erect as long as possible. But even if I was reduced to crawling, I would look people straight in the eye. I would not stare vacantly into space.

My name was called. My apprehension grew as I removed my upper clothing, draped myself in a tent-sized gown and walked to radiation room 1. Two technicians conversed, ignoring my presence. I was laid on a table with a grid in the center. Over me hung a huge machine. One technician bared the left half of my chest. She stretched out my left arm and ordered me to grasp a dowel to keep my arm steady. I was grateful when the other technician rolled a towel and propped it under my bicep for support. The inscrutable doctor glided in. The room lights were dimmed so that the treatment could be set up, guided by the light from the machine called a linear accelerator. Icily, the doctor directed the table to be raised . . . lowered . . . to the left . . . to the right. The younger technician responded clumsily in confusion. The second one said, "Remember, you move the table opposite of the way you want the light to move."

The clumsy technician's language was punctuated with incorrect verbs. "I seen it over there," she said as she pointed to the lead block the doctor asked for. I fought viewing her as a "typical dumb blonde." My life rested in her hands. The thought frightened me.

The doctor instructed her impatiently, as one would teach an inattentive child. "You will radiate in two stages. First the left super clavicular field"—she ran her finger along my collarbone—"and then the internal mammary field," she said, pointing to the sternum area.

The technician began to mark me on a spot the doctor directed.

The doctor stopped her. "That's not the way," she said.

"It's the way they taught us in school," the young blonde insisted.

"You're not in school." The doctor demonstrated a technique that eliminated unnecessary marks on the skin. Then she explained how to align the machine with the points she had marked and warned the technicians to use a lead block to screen my trachea so that I would not develop soreness or difficulty in swallowing.

The two technicians and the doctor left the room. The lights were flipped on. The door swished behind them.

From directly above me, through the intercom built into the arm of the machine, came the order "lie still, Mrs. Britton," followed by a whirring motor and a flashing light as my body was pelted with invisible rays. Time seemed to stand still.

The technicians and the doctor returned. The radiation therapist supervised as I was readjusted so that the procedure could be repeated. Once more I tensed in anticipation as the technicians left and I waited for the click and whir of the machine. But once more I felt nothing. Relieved, I sat up and slid the gown back over my shoulders. The technicians returned to lower the table and help me down.

As I was leaving the room, the technician admonished, "Don't wash this area until your treatments are completed."

"What would happen?" I asked, expecting a medical phenomenon.

"You would wash off the marks. We use washable marker."

The tension was broken. I began to giggle.

* * *

Before traveling to an afternoon appointment in Greenville with Dr. Coulter, Genny and I called the school to arrange Kris's early dismissal so that she could ride with us. The secretary said, "Oh, while I have you on the line, I'll get Mr. Soleman. He just mentioned that he wanted to talk to you."

Only a few moments passed until the dean spoke. "Mrs. Britton? I have several things I want you to know about your return to work." And then he began like a recorded message. I could not bring myself to interrupt him for any but perfunctory responses.

"First, I want to state that before I'll consider allowing you to teach, you must have a written doctor's release. This is mandatory."

I had never had an extended illness, so I didn't know if this was usual procedure for a nonphysical job such as teaching, but I said, "Of course, if you want one, there is no problem. I'm on my way to the doctor right now."

Not acknowledging my comments, he whirred on. "Second, I will agree to having your tenth-period class covered, but you must alternate days with the current substitute teacher. You may teach a maximum of three days a week. And of course you realize that there will be an appropriate salary adjustment for your shortened days."

He continued his monolog without pausing. "Also I expect you to be in school to observe your classes the day before your return."

In total disbelief, I stared at the wall in front of me. Without the time or energy for arguing, I simply stammered, "I will be in tomorrow to talk to you about the details. I must go now."

I hung up, visibly shaken. "What on earth is wrong?" Genny asked.

"I can't believe what I just heard." I reviewed the dean's position. "I thought that with my established reputation he'd be pleased that I want to return. Instead it looks as if I'm going to have to battle for my job."

"Don't worry about it now, Janet. Maybe there is a simple solution."

I avoided the dean when we picked up Kris from school, and I tried to push scheduling problems out of my mind so that I could concentrate on eliciting Dr. Coulter's opinion of the radiation therapist's treatment plan—especially her recommendation of subsequent chemotherapy.

* * *

Anticipating a hectic day, I slept until the last possible minute. That day Nancy was taking me first to a department store to be fitted for a prosthesis, then to my second radiation appointment, and finally to school to talk to the dean about my return to work.

The representative from Reach for Recovery had highly recommended Maline in this department store as a discreet fitter of prostheses. Following her suggestions to wear a tight-fitting, vertically striped top and to take a friend to check the fit, I felt well prepared for my shopping trip. I had both the stripes and the friend.

Nancy and I browsed in the lingerie department while we waited for Maline to finish with a customer. Strolling past see-through gowns, lace underpants and black strapless bras, I recalled my embarrassment at shopping for my first training bra. Again I felt I might be overcome by the preteen giggles. But I had determined to be coolly sophisticated. With great dignity, I introduced myself as Janet Britton and said I was scheduled to be fitted for a prosthesis.

Maline launched into action. Efficiently, she steered me back to a fitting room, dramatically inserted a key and with a flourish ushered me in. Not breaking her perpetual motion, she tiptoed back out, furtively securing the door. Momentarily I was alone in the cubbyhole. I heard shuffling and the key being reinserted. She pushed the door open with her hip and joggled in, in her 48D, balancing a pile of boxes. Even before catching her breath, she leaned forward to intensify the impending sales pitch. "I have a nice little bra here that will be just perfect for you." She dangled it by the straps just two inches from my nose. I took a deep breath and tried to appear discriminating.

Concentrating on the swinging bra in her left hand, I was shocked by her right hand darting out to unbutton my blouse as she said, "Let me see what size you are."

I blinked in disbelief. Maintaining my icy sophistication, I stepped back, stayed her with a glance, and throatily asserted, "I'll do that, thank you." Then hurriedly I fumbled with the buttons to disrobe before she felt compelled to aid me further.

I tried to shake off my first impressions of this pudgy little woman who shook her streaked gray head condescendingly as to a child who needed coddling. Regaining my composure, I hung my blouse on the hook and turned to face her stare.

"Oh, what's wrong with your neck?" She peered down her nose through her trifocals.

"Those are the markings for my radiation treatments. They must stay."

Automatically she moved to unsnap my bra for me. Just as automatically I shrank from her and struggled with the clasp myself. Hanging my bra with my blouse, I became conscious of my nakedness—my vulnerability.

Maline scrutinized me openly while engaging in small talk. "Who was your surgeon?"

"Dr. Coulter from Greenville."

"He did a really neat job." Again I heard the standard comment on my scar. "You're rather young for a mastectomy, aren't you? But of course they do such a good job any more treating . . . your problem."

I had to smile at her near error of pronouncing that taboo word *cancer*.

Following Reach for Recovery's suggestion, I asked for a bra with a pocket. But Maline insisted the bra she had selected was perfect. (Besides, her store didn't carry a bra with a pocket!) When I agreed to her choice, she shuffled another pile of boxes and said, "I have several sizes and designs of prosthesis here."

I avoided the avalanche of styles by telling her I'd been advised to ask for "the weighted one that's flesh colored." She still felt compelled to subject me to her polished sales pitch on "our best-selling item." Then she instructed me, "Place this circle toward the arm." She rearranged the prosthesis in my bra, ordered me to re-dress, and then stood shifting impatiently. As I scrutinized my image in the mirror, she called Nancy in to see the finished look.

"My left side seems larger than my right," I said.

As unaffected by my opinion as the mother of ten is by a child's whim, Maline brushed my hesitancy aside. "It looks perfect to me," she said. She turned to Nancy, who stood in the door of the dressing room, and asked, "Doesn't she look nice and natural to you?"

I waited for Nancy's honest appraisal. She confirmed my view that the prosthesis was larger than my natural side or "lopsided or something."

Maline ignored our inexpert opinions and collected her boxes. Behind her, Nancy gestured vehemently to encourage me to be aggressive. With determination, I insisted, "Besides it's too heavy on my shoulder."

Maline turned and spoke slowly and distinctly, as to a slow learner. "Of course it's heavy. That is its selling feature. That prevents your bra from riding up. You just need to adjust the strap so that the prosthesis is higher—like your other side."

Her hand darted out and hoisted the strap until I felt as if I could rest my chin on the prosthesis. Doggedly I maintained that the prosthesis was the wrong size. Nancy squirmed, trying to contain her amusement and frustration.

Maline was unperturbed. "Well, to add a little fullness to your natural side, you can use some of this lamb's wool that you have packed in the pocket of the bra you wore here." Efficiently, she stuffed. "There, do you like that better?"

I tried to make her understand that I was buying a prosthesis so that I wouldn't have to stuff my bra. She didn't seem to be hearing me. I felt as if I should lean over so she could read my lips. She was positive that I would be very satisfied with the fitting once I got used to the idea of a prosthesis. I felt as though I were trying to hold back a tidal wave with a wall made of popsicle sticks. At last I conceded, not wanting to be labeled a neurotic mastectomy patient. Further argument seemed futile.

Nonplused, Maline marked the bill "surgical" as she incessantly chattered about insurance problems until Nancy and I managed to steal away.

On the way to the car, I asked Nancy, "Am I walking tilted?"

She hesitated only slightly before shrugging her shoulders and trying to assure me that I looked "just fine."

I remembered the Bible's instruction to look for the good in all situations. I figured this was a perfect test of my obedience. My brow furrowed until I found it. "I always wondered what it would be like to have a sagging breast. Now at last I have one."

Nancy and I let out our suppressed giggles as we drove from

the department store to an uneventful second radiation treatment.

* * *

As Nancy turned the car toward the school, my hopes mounted
that my return to teaching would go smoothly.

I climbed the stairs and found the sub, who spoke enthusiastically about discontinuing work. I explored her reaction to the
plan of our teaching on alternate days. She was baffled and said
she would not agree to be tied down to such a schedule. Apparently the scheme had not originated with her.

As I was about to descend the steps, the superintendent rushed
up, gushing excitedly, and invited me into his office. I used
the opportunity to ask his opinion of my teaching alternate days.
He said he had heard nothing of the plan, but was sure that it
was meant to ease my transition back to work—to *protect* me
from overdoing.

"Since sick days are taken at the employee's discretion, I don't
have to agree to stay home when I'm well, do I?" I inquired innocently.

"Of course not," he answered. Then he disclosed that the dean
had expressed concern about my returning to teach before I was
able to do my job properly. "I explained that you are a reasonable
woman and that if we told you we felt you were no longer competent, you would willingly go back on sick leave."

I paused, counting to ten. "I hope you know that if I weren't
capable of teaching no one would have to tell me. I have too much
pride to return if I can't do a good job."

He did not respond. Next I tentatively probed his stand on Mr.
Soleman's request that I observe my classes the day before my
first day of work. I didn't mention how demeaned I felt by Mr.
Soleman's attitude, as if cancer made me incapable of making wise
decisions about my own health or profession. The superintendent
seemed surprised at the dean's request.

The super's responses bolstered my confidence. I turned to
Dean Soleman's office, determined to avoid confrontation while
firmly defending my position. I tried a positive approach. I smiled

and began, "The substitute and I just talked. She will be finished with the current units tomorrow. I will be back to school on Thursday. She said she will gladly substitute if I find it necessary to be absent."

Mr. Soleman gave no indication of noticing that I was ignoring his requests to teach every other day and spend a day in observation before my return.

* * *

Wednesday night I squeezed my eyes tightly and practiced my routine of proven sleep-inducing methods, but I only managed to doze fitfully. Although I had always been addicted to the snooze button, this day I popped out of bed forty-five minutes early.

Rex quietly beamed as I dressed. The children's reactions were not so contained. They bounced in and out of our bedroom, talking nonstop. Their voices were several tones higher than usual. Kris even gave me an extra hug.

My classroom was piled with the empty boxes that the paperbacks had been packed in during the summer, with almost five months' mail, and with general clutter. Bare walls stared back at me. In spite of my weakness, I could not stand to teach in such a desolate room for even a day. I enlisted the help of my first-period class. Enthusiastically the students pitched in. As I directed them, they scurried like a colony of ants shouldering their bundles. In just one period the room became more familiar, more cozy.

Between first and second period, Kris darted in. "How are you doing? Do you feel all right?" she asked breathlessly.

I convinced her that I was just fine.

As she turned to fly down the hall, she whispered, "I love you. I'm glad you're here."

Other students reinforced her encouragement. Scribbled notes were dropped on my desk by my previous students: "Glad you're back!" New students greeted me warmly: "I really enjoy class now that you're teaching!" and "The kids were right when they said you were an O.K. teacher." Their reception strengthened me. Love and purpose—what more could I ask for?

As previously arranged, my professor arrived to speak to my

senior English classes. Presenting me with a terrarium and a card from several of the Y.S.U. English faculty, she quietly said, "We wanted to celebrate with you your return to the classroom." As she encouraged my students to hone their writing skills before attending college, I basked in the respect of my graduate school professors and my students. But my pride was dampened by the fact that the administration was hesitant to accept me back as a competent professional. Having to prove to the administration that I remained a master teacher seemed like a huge task.

After my classes, I stumbled to the front of the school where a friend waited to drive me to my radiation treatment. I brimmed with information about school. I wanted to share the events of my day. But I was too weary. My head leaned heavily on the headrest, and I soon slept.

By the time I was delivered home, my left shoulder throbbed from the deep groove dug by my bra strap. And in spite of the gauze padding which protected the graft site, the constant pressure had generated a dull ache. As soon as I pulled myself through the door, I tossed the prosthesis onto the kitchen counter, flopped onto a kitchen chair and dialed my mother to complain about the weight of the prosthesis.

Mom persuaded me to be refitted. I called Maline and explained my problem. "I've never had a complaint before," she insisted, "but by all means, do come in tomorrow." Her tone of voice made me feel neurotic.

When I returned to the department store, I felt like a child slinking back home after running away from a scolding.

Maline bustled and bristled as she set out to "see what the problem is." And then, suddenly, as if she had made an independent discovery, she said, "Why, I believe this prosthesis is the wrong size. Someone must have picked up the wrong box." In response to this sudden insight, she arranged a smaller prosthesis in my bra.

The new prosthesis filled the left side naturally and comfortably. "Now that looks more like me," I said.

* * *

The next morning Renae, bounding into our bedroom, halted and stared curiously as I adjusted the prosthesis. "What's that thing, Mom?"

"It's called a prosthesis. It makes this side of my bra look the same as the other side."

"Why do you need it?"

"Well, remember I told you that the doctor had to cut off the bad cells in my breast? If I didn't put this thing in my bra, this side would be flat and the other side would stick out and my blouses would look funny."

"Oh," she said, apparently satisfied, for she launched immediately into a story about the boy in school who stole her last pencil the day before. I found a pencil for her to take to school and she skipped back downstairs.

Rex, too, quickly learned about the value of my prosthesis. I had discussed its potential. "I'm looking forward to being sexually harassed. When the man makes his move, I'll whip out my prosthesis and say, 'Oh, so you want to pinch and feel breasts? Well, here. Enjoy yourself.' That should scare him away."

But I didn't wait to be propositioned to experiment with my new weapon. One night as I lay exhausted on the couch, Rex began to tease me. When I threatened to retaliate, he boasted that he was safe since I was obviously too tired to handle him. In one quick motion, I reached into my blouse, grabbed the prosthesis and zinged it at his head. He ducked and it hit with a thud on the wall behind him. His eyes popped wide open, and then he started chuckling. "A man isn't safe around you, even if you do appear defenseless."

I agreed. "You have to be extra careful now. I may not have energy to jump up and attack, but I have a new secret weapon."

* * *

At first I couldn't believe that the administration might actually prefer that I stay on sick leave. But their attitude was made clear on Friday, my second day back to school, when the dean appeared at my door inquiring about how I felt.

"Oh, I'm doing just fine," I answered naively.

"Aren't you pretty tired, teaching two days in a row?" He stared at me intensely.

Slightly wary, I repeated that I was fine, adding, "Even if I have to sleep every moment I'm not at school, I'll make sure I have enough rest to do my job well."

The dean's mask did not drop. He stared, unblinking.

"Anyway, I won't hurt anyone else. Cancer isn't contagious, you know."

My obvious attempt at humor engendered no response. His deadpan expression did not alter. He turned, without further comment, and disappeared downstairs. I gazed after him, trying to understand him.

Later that day it was explained to me that the dean had wanted the substitute to work alternating days so that she could keep abreast of my classes. "Qualified substitutes in English are hard to find. We must keep her busy in case we need her later this year."

"I don't think there'll be a need for a permanent sub at least until next school year," I said, smiling ingratiatingly. Inwardly I boiled.

The situation intensified. The superintendent informed me that if I were allowed to leave without a penalty, then other teachers could also demand to leave early. Allowing me to go for radiation therapy was a dangerous precedent.

I lashed out. "It would be a precedent only for teachers who have cancer and are going for radiation treatments. Hopefully there won't be many of those."

He did not respond. I had been dismissed. Mutely, I conceded and made plans to go on half-day sick leave.

I became defensive. My mind dwelt on the programs I had initiated in my eight years of working in this school district, on the summers I'd spent improving my professional skills, and on the grant programs I had written. I had invested hundreds of hours of my own time in these projects. It was inconceivable to me that now, when I requested twenty-two days of a shortened schedule, the district would quibble. Certainly I had always been a financial asset.

But I had to acknowledge that in the administration's view

my ability to remain an asset was very much in question. Dad had found employers hesitant to employ anyone with a record of cancer. Perhaps attitudes had not progressed much in the last fifteen years, even among the college educated.

My schedule was changed four times in the next few weeks. I kept reminding myself that I was supposedly dealing with educated and rational men who surely understood that my physical disability was not an intellectual impairment. I fought believing that a cancer phobia was involved in their decisions.

I felt driven to be productive. Then, just as he spoke to Martha, I heard Christ speak to me, "Janet, Janet, you are worried and upset about many things, but only one thing is important."

"But the administration is treating me as if I were dead or at least a debit. And I've worked hard to develop my expertise as a teacher. All anyone has to do to verify my efficiency is observe my classroom." I continued petulantly, "It's just like when Dad had cancer. No one wanted to have him work for them."

God patiently listened.

"This is the first time after all these years that I've ever needed help. Instead of help, I get attacked. I'm treated like an enemy or at least a stranger."

"Pray for those that despitefully use you and persecute you."

"You must be kidding!"

"No, child." God shook his head tenderly.

"Oh, I give up. I thought you had work for me at school," I huffed in exasperation. "But thy will be done."

"That's right, Janet. I give you the good works to do."

"Well, I'm learning, Father. This time it only took me weeks to accept your will. My acceptance of Dad's death took months. I am growing, aren't I?"

"Yes, child. You are getting to be a big girl."

The next day I was informed that the administration had reconsidered its position. They asked if, during the final two weeks of my radiation treatments, I would return to the original plan of leaving early.

After three weeks of confusion, my schedule was finally set.

* * *

The routine of my 2:30 appointments seldom varied. I rushed from school to be chauffeured by a friend to Southside Hospital. The first two weeks I rode to the parking deck and then walked back to the hospital entrance. But as I became progressively more exhausted, I was delivered directly to the outpatient surgery entrance where I shuffled through the automatic opening doors and slumped into an orange plastic chair until my driver joined me.

The first weeks I had insisted on asserting my strength by descending the twenty-six steps, but as the radiation's effect grew, exhaustion's weight forced me to succumb to riding the elevator down one floor where we wound through the bowels of the building—past vending machines, offices, the entrance to physical therapy and the dental clinic until finally, directly in front of us, loomed a set of double doors labeled Radiation Therapy.

We were guided through this labyrinth of halls by orange signs which hung from the beige walls like signs on an interstate. The clicking of our heels on the glossy tile echoed as we passed Examining Room 1, Examining Room 2 and No Admittance. We made a final right turn through the entrance of an L-shaped room divider which shielded patients from the world's gaze. To the left of the entrance the receptionist hid, safely shielded behind a glass window whose sill held a legal pad on which patients signed in. A skeletal coat rack gestured menacingly at me each day as I selected a turquoise vinyl seat and an outdated ladies' magazine from the pile on an end table. Ironically, each one seemed to contain an article on cancer. A sign on the wall warned us all not to smoke, although I couldn't help thinking that it was probably too late for most occupants of the room to worry about that now. The solitary link to the outside world was the pay phone hanging on the wall.

A single picture adorned the barren walls. Every day I would stare at the sad gray kitten painted on the solid black background. The only brightness was in the blocks, one red and one green, on which the kitten rested its paws. I was penetrated by the eyes of that kitten. Seemingly filled with tears, they reflected the expressions on the faces of the patients—tired, melancholy, distracted.

An FM station played softly to cover the silence. The paging of a doctor or the announcement of a meeting for the hospital staff frequently interrupted the music.

I talked to God. "Is this the place David meant when he talked about the valley of the shadow of death?"

"Not exactly, but that phrase seems to fit, doesn't it?"

"But you are with me?"

"Yes, my child, so fear no evil!" I clung to my Father.

When the receptionist called my name, I trudged to one of the dressing cubicles—the bathroomlike stalls with beige metal doors which opened to reveal a bench and a clothes hook. I grabbed the top gown from the pile on the bench, wrapped it like a sheet around me and then waited in the hall on one of the two red chairs by the scales. I memorized the clutter on the counters which held the closed-circuit monitors—a coffee cup labeled Bayer, a telephone, several filled ashtrays, Kleenex and postcards and pictures from patients. I watched as one technician monitored the patient on the screen and the other recorded the dosage administered. And I listened to the boisterous tone that the blonde technician, Patty, adopted when speaking to patients. I wondered if she knew that cancer is not symptomized by hearing loss.

When it was my turn, I passed the "Caution Radiation" sign on the door of room 1. There the two technicians and I performed our daily ritual as we conversed about children, husbands, the weather, our jobs. The procedure became so automatic that the three of us played our parts effortlessly.

I stepped up on a stool, lay on the table and removed my gown from my left shoulder. One technician turned off the room lights. The other raised the table. Together they aligned the light from the machine with the markings on my neck and shoulder area. The technician flicked the room lights back on and the door swung shut behind them. Through the intercom on the machine's arm I'd hear the instructions, "Don't move." Whir. Click. The minute passed. The linear accelerator switched off.

My tender chest and underarm ached from the extended position, but not from the thousands of rays which penetrated their tissues. The technicians returned and realigned the machine with the marks on my breastbone. The process was repeated. The second time they returned to the room, they lowered the table. Each day one of the technicians automatically reached out to assist me to the floor. Each day I tactfully ignored the hand. "See you tomorrow," Patty would yell. I would subtract one from the number of treatments that remained.

Just as I thought I had become hardened to this routine, a remark slipped from a friend and forced me to observe the scene with fresh vision. "I'd never do this," she mumbled, shaking her head. I saw the marks, the vacant stares, the broken hair; I touched my own neck covered by a scarf, and I understood her remark. But remembering my own father's illness, I wanted her to understand my choice. "You would if you had young children. My family must experience no guilt."

She looked bewildered. I dropped the subject.

*   *   *

November 14, the day of my last radiation treatment, Rex mentioned that he planned to drive to Youngstown to buy vinyl siding for an extra job he and a friend had contracted. I suggested that he stop at the school on his way to take me for my treatment. He was hesitant. I wheedled him. After thirteen years of marriage, I knew how to convince him. He grumbled, but agreed.

When he arrived, I climbed into his pickup, deliberately cheerful. "How's my lover?" I asked and gave him a big kiss.

His frozen expression did not thaw. He grunted a response. I chatted, pretending to be oblivious to his mood. I tried to coax him out of his depression. I felt as if I were on a first date with the most popular boy in school whom I was trying to impress. But I had the feeling this date was going to be a gigantic flop.

A couple of blocks from the hospital, Rex broke his silence. "You know I didn't want to come."

"But, Rex, I want you to know what I'm talking about when I mention the staff and the procedure of my radiation treatments.

It's all much simpler than you must imagine." He remained unconvinced.

That day there was no waiting since I was several minutes late. I felt a twinge of gratitude that no obviously ill patients were sitting there.

"Come back with me, honey," I ordered. He obeyed. I introduced him to the two technicians who had shared my past five weeks. They showed Rex the radiation machine, and he watched while they set it for my treatment. The three of them left, and the technicians had him observe the monitor while I was being pelted with radiation. He returned with them for the second setting. By then he was joking with them. I felt like hugging them for their kindness to him.

"You have to stay for your weekly appointment with the doctor now," the technician reminded me. She escorted us to a vacant examining room adjacent to the treatment rooms.

Rex shuffled impatiently. At last the doctor arrived with a nurse at her side. I introduced them to Rex, but the doctor barely acknowledged his presence. She glanced at my chart and said, "I see your series has been completed." Then she started to leave. "I want to see you again in three months to check for anything new."

Obviously confused, Rex blurted, "What are you looking for?"

She kept walking. She ignored his question. The nurse looked at her receding back and then at Rex. Rex repeated, "What is she looking for?"

In a professionally delicate position, the nurse replied flippantly, "I guess you'll just have to come back with your wife in three months to find out."

Rex bristled. "I knew I shouldn't have come," he said flatly.

I dressed and again he asked the receptionist, "Why does Janet have to make another appointment? I thought this was the last one."

"The doctor will want to make sure there are no new lumps under the arm or around the scar tissue."

"But Janet had the lymph nodes taken out so that there wouldn't be lumps under her arm."

The receptionist was confused. I intervened. "She really doesn't know, honey."

We left immediately. Rex erected a wall between us so I couldn't hurt him further. His jaw remained clenched all the way home. No wonder Rex is so defensive, I thought. Over and over he has been cornered by the medical community—unable to defend himself or his wife, unable even to have his reasonable questions answered.

Chemical Warfare

CHEMO—THE WORD CONJURED UP NIGHTMARE IMAGES OF THIN, bald "victims," riddled by infections and puking out their guts. How could I passively subject myself to such treatment? I would have to be convinced that the therapy was essential and life-saving.

The day Dr. Nath mentioned chemotherapy, I dashed to my surgeon's office and attacked him before he could close the examining room door. "Why didn't you tell me I'd need more than radiation? The radiation therapist wants me to begin chemotherapy as soon as the radiation cycle is completed. You never warned me."

Patiently, Dr. Coulter explained that in the tumor board's discussion of my case, there was total agreement on the advantages of the oophorectomy and radiation therapy. But there was some disagreement on the necessity of chemotherapy. He had decided to rely on the recommendation of the doctors in Youngstown for that final decision.

Succinctly, he summarized the two main schools of thought. "The first, to which I've usually subscribed, believes in waiting until there is a recurrence, usually seen in the bone scans, before beginning chemotherapy. The second, the current trend, prefers beginning treatments immediately to avoid a recurrence. And current research on the two methods shows no appreciable difference in survival rates."

Given those options, I had determined to refuse chemotherapy and to take my chances. After all, without chemotherapy I would soon regain strength. Dad had lived over two years without any symptoms before his last recurrence. That time would be invaluable to my husband and children. Chemo would postpone returning to normal life for over a year.

But Dr. Coulter urged me not to make a final decision until I had consulted with the chemotherapist. Cynically, I thought, "Of course he'll say I should start the treatments. It's his field. He'd have to believe in what he's doing." But I decided it wouldn't hurt to at least talk to the chemotherapist. Besides I was curious to find out what his reasoning would be.

November 17, the Monday following my last radiation treatment, Mom and I stepped into the medical annex of Northside Hospital in Youngstown. A hall lined with chairs introduced us to the department of oncology and hemotology—the study of tumors and blood diseases.

As on my first visit to Southside's radiation department, I concentrated on talking to my companion rather than observing my soon-to-be-familiar surroundings.

Mom stood and followed me into a conference room at the nurse's call for "Mrs. Britton." Dr. Bhatti—a short, round-faced, almond-skinned man with compassionate, honest eyes—introduced himself and noted my referral from the radiation therapists. Immediately he launched into questions about my medical history. The list of diseases stretched on and on. "No, I haven't. No, I haven't," was my standard response. No, no previous surgeries except for a tubal ligation and vein stripping after Neil was born. The irony of the situation struck me. "I guess this isn't the place to say it," I said, "but I'm really a very healthy person."

The doctor's eyes twinkled. He asked his concluding question, "Do you have an appetite?"

That was a difficult question to answer truthfully. "No—but I eat a lot. Does that make sense?"

His puffy cheeks crinkled. "Yes, it makes perfect sense to me."

I decided I liked this man. I felt free to be open with him. "I want to state clearly that I am here to be convinced that chemotherapy at this time is necessary. My surgeon said that statistics show the same results whether I begin chemotherapy now or wait until a recurrence. Is he right? Or is there evidence to support beginning therapy now?"

Dr. Bhatti built an intense, logical case for his position. "First I'll tell you that I don't believe in making guesses about life spans because no one can determine how a body will react. There are too many variables—physical and emotional. We are investigators. We have no cure for cancer, so I cannot promise to cure you. Perhaps some people would say that our statistics are not impressive. Many of our patients eventually die of cancer. But we can promise our patients an extended life. A year or two may not look impressive on a graph, but a year or two of quality life is significant to the individual and to the people who love that individual."

He paused and I acknowledged that I certainly agreed with that view.

He smiled and continued. "The purpose of chemotherapy is to destroy cancer cells. If we don't succeed, there will eventually be a recurrence. But even if we don't destroy all the cancer cells, chemotherapy definitely will lower the population so that the growth of a detectable mass is retarded. We buy time. It may be enough time for scientists to find the cure for the disease. Or it may just mean a longer life for you. Sometimes we get lucky and destroy the complete population, and the cancer never recurs."

I considered this information before I said, "But the radiation therapist used the term *prophylactic* chemotherapy. In other words, no one is sure that I won't be fine anyway even if I have no more treatments."

The doctor's black eyes fired. "We are constantly instructing doctors not to use the word *prophylactic*. It's inappropriate. We don't treat something that doesn't exist. If there were significant doubts about the spread of your disease, we would not schedule you for the treatments." And he went over the same facts that the radiation therapist had referred to a month and a half previously. I had had a positive node. There had been metastasis to my lymphatic system. And the lesion was medially located. Involvement of the central lower quadrant gave the worst prognosis. The tumor was fast growing. I was only thirty-three. And I had had positive estrogen receptors which increased the likelihood of a good response to hormonal treatment.

I stopped his lecture. "But I had an oophorectomy. I thought that the removal of my ovaries was supposed to stop the growth of any cells that had spread. Without estrogen the cells will die."

"The oophorectomy is a logical response to the positive estrogen receptors in patients who are still menstruating. But we don't have statistics yet to prove the effectiveness of the surgery."

"Then I had it for no reason."

"No, an oophorectomy is part of a complete program of attack."

I tried to digest all the material we were discussing.

"But I'm still not sure that it's necessary to begin chemotherapy now. What answer would you give to the surgeon who says that the therapy will work just as well later if a mass does eventually occur on the bone or lungs?"

Confidently Dr. Bhatti said, "A detectable mass is composed of millions of cells. It is logical that we have a better chance of destroying the population while the number of cells is still microscopic."

He cleared his throat, then added, "I also believe that it is psychologically cruel to wait until there is a mass. The damage to the psyche of a recurrence is significant. We know positive attitudes improve quality of life, so it is important to protect the patient emotionally as well as physically. We are practicing physicians, but we are also researchers affiliated with larger groups carrying on treatment and research in other parts of the country. We pool results of different approaches and base our therapy on those which are found to be most helpful. And the best evidence we have now points to your undergoing immediate therapy."

The doctor's honest appraisal of the facts, his direct and human approach, his respect for me as an individual, swayed me to his position. I made no protest when he concluded, "I will schedule you to begin therapy a week from today. I will calculate the maximum dosage that your body will allow. We need to use an aggressive treatment to fight an aggressive disease."

The nurse weighed and measured me so that the doctor could compute my body surface area and prescribe the dosage of methotrexate (MTX) and 5-Flurouracil (5-FU) for the outlined protocol. I would be scheduled for two injections a month. The day of my first injection, I would also begin taking Cytoxan pills morning and evening for two weeks. One week from the first injection, I would receive a second injection of the 5-FU and MTX mixture. Four weeks from the first injection I would return to begin the cycle once more. The twenty-eight-day cycle would continue for at least twelve months. When all the lab tests were back, I would also begin taking four pills a day, for a minimum of two years, of a hormone-blocking agent called Tamoxifen.

Twelve months—one year of weakness and nausea. How could I voluntarily subject myself to this program now? How could I compound my weakness by adding the effects of chemotherapy to those of surgery and radiation? I knew that within three months the effects of radiation would dissipate and I would regain my strength. Why not enjoy that strength until a recurrence forced me into chemotherapy?

But my mind replayed the doctor's comment. "At your age you have more years to gain." He was right. I was gambling one year of debilitation to gain two years, or perhaps even a normal life span, another forty or fifty years. But what if I lost the gamble? Why should I give up a year of strength and comparative health if I had but a few valuable years left? With my normal strength, I could accomplish a lot in twelve months—especially in the training of my children. But weakened and struggling to function, I could do little valuable work.

The pros and cons battered my mind as I left the hospital.

* * *

I waited until Rex and I were alone in bed that night before discussing Dr. Bhatti's position.

I sensed a warning buzzer moments before Rex exploded. "Chemotherapy? Twenty-five days of radiation? I thought the oophorectomy was to be the end. Why didn't Dr. Coulter tell us what to expect?"

I pointed out that the surgeon had told us radiation would be necessary.

"But not at the beginning." Rex leaped from the bed and paced around the room. "First he says just to have the lump removed and that will be the end of it. Then he says just have a mastectomy and everything will be fine. Then he says if you have another surgery you will be fine. Then he tells you to go to a radiation therapist and you will be fine. Now you're told to have chemotherapy and that will take care of everything."

I pointed out that cancer is difficult to treat and that doctors go only a step at a time so that the patient won't become discouraged. But Rex said he preferred knowing everything from the beginning. In his frustration, he went on, "What no one will say out loud is that you'll never be fine. This whole thing will never end. You'll never be the woman I married."

That statement stung. "I thought you were the one who didn't want me to have a reconstruction," I retaliated.

Rex shook his head. "I knew you wouldn't understand. I'm not talking about the surgery. Do you think I married you for your bra size? I told you your breast isn't important, and I meant it. I'm saying you'll never be able to do the things we used to. You're always going to be tired. This illness will never end."

As Rex calmed down, I heated up. "What do you want me to do? Die? Would that make you happy? Then all of this would end."

Rex raged once more. "There you go saying something stupid

again. I don't know why I bother talking to you. You never understand."

He flopped back onto our bed. We lay with stiff backs separating us. Both of us were hurt and scared.

*   *   *

The next evening when I returned from school I overheard Rex talking on the phone. "Do you think they'd take $40,000 for it? [Pause.] My price is firm. You know that this farm is worth every penny."

I couldn't believe my ears. He was talking about selling our home! I tried not to overreact. I vowed I would not repeat the mistake of attacking as I had the night before.

"Who were you talking to, honey?" I asked, smiling nonchalantly.

"Edwina."

"Why?"

"Oh, I just had a few questions I wanted to ask her."

"About what?"

"Oh, nothing important."

"What do you consider unimportant?" I prodded carefully.

"I just was asking her about real-estate prices."

"Why?"

"She told me a while ago that she had several people interested in buying our farm. A fifty-acre farm is a premium deal—especially for people coming from Cleveland. It's just the right size for hobby farming. I wanted to see if she still has a buyer."

Tentatively I asked where he was planning to move. The house he had in mind was within the village limits. I reminded him that we had moved from town because we thought the country was a better environment for our children. But he pointed out that living in town would be more convenient for me. He built to his major point—we ought to sell our place because we might not be able to continue to afford the farm. "That's eventually," I argued. "We don't have to sell now. Let's wait until there's no other choice."

In spite of my arguments, for the next few days real estate kept cropping up in conversations. Outwardly I remained calm. Inwardly my tension mounted. What I didn't tell Rex was that I felt he was admitting defeat. He was acting on the belief that I would soon be too ill to function. He had lost faith in my recovery.

"Father, Rex is so fatalistic. I don't have the energy to move. And, besides, I don't want to. Help!"

"I've promised never to allow you to be tempted more than you can bear."

I protested, "But I'm never sure if that means you'll change the circumstances or just give me strength to bear more!"

"Either way my strength is sufficient for you."

I didn't have to wait long to understand my Father's answer. A few evenings later Rex's friend Freeman told me Rex's reasons for wanting to move. Rex felt guilty that I had to teach to help pay the mortgage. Hesitantly Freeman explained, "Rex wants to make it possible for you to resign and just be a housewife. He's worried that you're pushing yourself too hard. I think he has a point."

I felt I had been given an opportunity to convince Rex, through this proxy, of the psychological importance of my working. I took a deep breath and began to enumerate my reasons for working. "Paying for this farm doesn't force me to school. My own need for normal routine does. And teaching is not physically strenuous like housework. I can sit if I'm tired. Running a sweeper or scrubbing a floor exhausts me—my body isn't efficient. But my brain still is."

I also tried to point out the benefits to our children of my teaching. My failure to work would be a constant reminder that Mommy's sick. And I'd have the burden every day of transporting Kris to and from school and worrying about her skipping classes or smoking in the restroom. I saved my strongest argument until last: "I could waste months waiting to feel better. But I have to live my life today. The best medicine for me is normal routine and usefulness."

At the end of our conversation, I knew Freeman would act as my ally. I prayed he could make Rex accept my views; I couldn't.

* * *

I tingled expectantly as I stepped to the speaker's podium at a workshop at the seventieth annual convention of the National Council of Teachers of English. I had anticipated this moment since a professor arranged the invitation almost a year previously. So in spite of my illness, I refused to cancel out. Such an honor might never be repeated. Following Ginger, my friend who described an independent reading program based on one I had originally developed, I spoke on the growth of the writing program which had led to the writing lab in our high school. After my presentation, another friend demonstrated exercises for teaching sentence combining. I had arrived at Stouffer's Cincinnati Towers slightly intimidated by the notables scheduled for the program—a Harvard professor, a contemporary woman poet, several well-known fiction and textbook authors (we were billed as three high-school teachers with innovative ideas and techniques). But the audience responded positively to our presentation. During the discussion period which followed our three lectures, professors, high-school teachers and textbook representatives enthusiastically shared their opinions and asked our advice. When the session was over, people swarmed around us.

The Y.S.U. professors, impressed by our reception, suggested that we celebrate our success. I puffed, trying to keep up, as the group ran all over town ferreting out the perfect restaurant. When we found it, I collapsed into a plush seat, ordered steak and wild rice, and peacefully absorbed the conversations around me. Nodding assent and laughing at jokes, I concentrated on Gratia Murphy, the professor who had spoken to my classes the month before. As she discussed the novels of a scheduled conference speaker and entertained us with literary anecdotes, I ruminated on her obviously successful career as a professor.

Gratia's career and mine had similar beginnings. She had begun teaching in a small high school just twenty-five miles from my school district. Also the wife of a laborer, she had commuted to do her graduate work while rearing a daughter and a son. We had so much in common.

As I listened to her, my emotions tumbled. *I'm just tired,* I thought, but I knew there was more. I could not forget that I had just completed five weeks of radiation and was scheduled for my first chemotherapy injection on Monday when I returned from Cincinnati. I couldn't disregard the fact that I might never have the opportunity for a career like Gratia's. "When the children are graduated from high school, I will go to Cleveland for my Ph.D. and will still have twenty years to be a professor," I had always said. My illness sneered at that goal.

The line, "Only what's done for Christ will last," echoed piously through my mind. Rationally I knew that only the people I influenced had eternal value. "In a hundred years no one will know or care if I finished my graduate work. No one will even care what profession I had," I argued with myself. *But I want that satisfaction,* I thought. *Maybe achieving a degree isn't eternally important. But right now, I still want a successful career.* My emotions prepared to throw themselves onto the floor and kick their feet. I sat, despondent. To sustain life, bread and spinach may be more important body-builders than chocolate-covered cherries or banana splits. I could survive without the desserts. But my life would be less enjoyable without them, and I didn't want to give them up. That's how I felt about wanting to become a college professor.

I wanted to lash out. How could this invader body do this to me? I could accept its alternately freezing me and steam-cooking me, its nausea and dizziness even. But I could not accept its continual refusal to obey my commands. It would not compromise. It refused to follow the schedules I made. It mocked my efforts by demanding rest and flaunting its control. I was its prisoner. And the worst irony was that this body did not dabble in idle threats. It could kill me. On a whim it could destroy all my plans for family and career.

I determined to defy this body by finishing my work for my master's degree immediately. I would not delay the work until therapy was completed and risk losing the opportunity to graduate. Perhaps I'd never have a Ph.D. Maybe I'd never write my book. Maybe I'd never be a respected English professor. This body might foil all these plans. But, no matter if others believed I was foolish; I would be victorious in the battle to finish the M.A.

in English as I'd planned. Earlier in our trip Gratia had given me a depressing message from my adviser: Y.S.U. definitely would not accept the transfer of my five credits from Kent State. But with my new resolve, I refused to be discouraged any longer by this news. Somehow I would earn the credits to graduate the summer of 1981.

My mother's reaction to my decision was typical of the responses of my friends and family. She jerked up and with hands on hips demanded, "What do you mean, you're going to take graduate courses? Working and attending classes is difficult enough for a person who's well. How do you think you can handle that schedule when you're sick? Wait until you feel better."

"What if I never feel better?" I argued.

"Then it really doesn't matter in the long run, does it?"

I knew she was being logical, but I wouldn't back down. "It matters to me. I started and I'm finishing. This may be the strongest I'll be, so I'll not wait."

* * *

"Do you think I'm a fool too, Father?"

"Child, I give you good gifts—the desires of your heart."

"So if you're for me, no one can be against me?"

The heavenly Father held his pampered, spoiled child.

* * *

The Monday after Thanksgiving, the morning after our return from Cincinnati, Genny and I walked up to the entrance of the medical annex to my first chemotherapy treatment. As I passed a wobbly man, a fountain of green liquid spewed from his mouth. "No, not that!" I cried inwardly. I wanted to turn and run away, but I didn't—at least not physically. Instead I isolated myself emotionally. Barely perceiving events around me, I found myself in the examining room, my middle finger bandaged after the "finger stick" for my blood count and my top half draped in a stiff hospital gown. Almost before I registered Dr. Bhatti's presence in the room, the examination was ending. I forced myself to concentrate on his staccato statements.

"There are several effects of chemotherapy that you may have. Hair loss, mouth sores, nausea and vomiting, possible weight gain, and blood in the urine are some of them. Take no medication that contains aspirin. I recommend Tylenol for headache and Co-Tylenol for colds and flu symptoms. If you have any symptom that is unusual, call me immediately." He opened the door and said over his shoulder as he was leaving, "Get dressed and the nurse will be in shortly to give you your injection. Be sure to go to the lab for a blood test afterward."

I felt overwhelmed by the matter-of-fact listing of side effects. I questioned the wisdom of our decision to go ahead with chemotherapy.

"Come with me, Janet. My name is Norma." I followed the nurse into a large room with chaise longues, straight-backed chairs and Mayos, adjustable stands on which patients rest their arms for treatments. Norma gathered a tourniquet and syringes and was ready to begin my treatment. I delayed her.

"The doctor mentioned the possibility of blood in the urine. Why would I have that?"

"All major organs are affected by the medication," she explained. "The Cytoxan sometimes irritates the bladder. We nurses always try to stress that you should drink as much liquid as you can so that the chemical doesn't just lie in your bladder and crystalize."

"What about the hair loss? How serious is that with my medication?"

"You will notice much thinning, but most of our patients don't buy wigs." Maybe that was a small thing to worry about but I was relieved that I might escape looking like a cue ball. "Cytoxan and 5-FU affect the hair. You understand that whereas radiation is a localized treatment that only affects the area of treatment, chemotherapy is a systemic treatment designed to attack any fast-growing cell. There's a delicate balance between normal and abnormal cells. Cancer cells are extremely fast growing, but so are some normal cells such as the hair follicles, parts of the digestive tract and certain blood cells. Unfortunately a chemical will take some of the good cells, too. It doesn't know any better."

I told Norma that I still questioned the value of subjecting myself to a year's treatments—especially if I didn't ultimately survive.

Her compassionate eyes soothed me as she described working in a study at Case Western Reserve in Cleveland for two years where the protocol of an Italian doctor was researched. "In the two-year study there was a definite reduction in the mortality rate. We aren't sure that there still won't be many recurrences, but we know the therapy extends lives." She paused to let me ponder these facts.

"Will I be able to continue my work?"

"The side effects should be controllable. And we find that people who stay as active as possible respond best to treatment. We urge people to maintain as normal a schedule as they can."

Norma continued answering my questions for at least thirty minutes. Outwardly unconcerned about the time, she gave me her complete attention. Finally I decided that since I would ultimately consent to the treatment, I might as well not continue the stall tactics.

"We'll draw your blood here first instead of sending you to the lab," Norma said. "We use a smaller diameter needle than the lab, and we can simply transfer the vial and save you one puncture."

I thanked her for her thoughtfulness.

"It's not just that we want to save you discomfort. We also want to save your veins as long as we can." This factual statement reverberated ominously through my mind.

As she tightened the band on my arm, I sat with my head turned. She finished drawing blood and began injecting the chemo. Nausea was almost instantaneous. A metallic taste crept into my mouth.

"That taste. Is it psychological?" I asked Norma.

"No, it's a chemical reaction. Many patients complain of the taste."

I understood now why the hard candy was at the receptionist's window. I wanted to rush out to see if a piece would disguise the pollution of my saliva.

I had expected the first treatment to be mild. I figured the effects of the chemicals would build in intensity as the effects of radiation had. But I was wrong. I fought the nausea. I began to burp.

*   *   *

The week I began chemotherapy was memorable for a second reason. That Friday, the day after Thanksgiving, Rex and I received a phone call from Ron. "I wondered if I could stay a few days with you until I find a place to live up there," he said.

Rex and I both assured Ron that we always had plenty of room for a friend. He was welcome for as long as he wanted to stay. We understood that Ron was giving every penny possible to support Ann and the children and that he couldn't afford to continue doing that and pay rent too. In Virginia he had been living out of the back of his pickup camper to economize; the weather was getting much too cold for him to consider that in Ohio. But Ron was so proud. We must not allow him to feel that he was intruding. It would be difficult to convince him to stay with us for as long as he needed to.

Ron arrived the next day with all his possessions in the back of his pickup truck.

I directed him to unpack his clothes in Neil's room since it had a bunk bed. "Use the empty drawers for your things," I said, but he refused.

"No, I'll just put a few things in your basement until I find a place to rent."

Tall and lean, blond and tanned, quietly smiling, he carried his clothes to the basement and hung them on the clothesline. Clinging to the past, he had stored his toothbrush, razor and other toiletries in the small milk pail in which he had for years carried the family's milk from the barn. His most valued possession seemed to be his hope in returning his family to farm life. Animatedly, Ron unrolled the detailed house plans he had drawn. While managing his father's farm, Ron had contracted for an adjoining one hundred acres, just to be able to cultivate land he called his own. He hoped now to build a home on this land that could serve his family until he was able to purchase his father's dairy farm.

The plans Ron showed us were meticulous. For economy, the design was a pole structure, but as he flipped the sketches of the four stages, a small utility-type building mushroomed into an attractively bricked ranch-style home. His eyes gleamed as he talked.

Sunday morning after he arrived, I noticed that his bunk had not been slept in. A foam pad and sleeping bag were rolled neatly in the corner.

"Why didn't you sleep in the bed, Ron?" I inquired.

"I don't want to put you guys out any," he answered.

"The bed is empty," Rex argued. "You aren't putting anyone out." But Monday morning the bed still had not been used. Rex and I did not push the issue. We knew that if Ron was more comfortable about staying in our home sleeping on the floor, then it was best to say nothing more.

Ron was a man who not only planned but also put feet under those plans. That Monday while I taught and went for my second chemotherapy injection, he scurried about until he found a job with a local fertilizer dealer, a man he had known and patronized for years. To finance the first phase of his house, he put a "For Sale" sign on his new pickup and took back the almost worthless red rattletrap he had parked at his father's farm.

* * *

Each day after this second injection, I found it harder to keep going. My chest was heavy. I coughed. Of all times to get a cold, I thought. To fight off the cold before it developed into more, I stayed home from school Thursday. Although I slept all morning, my cough progressively worsened. I called Dr. Bhatti to see if he would prescribe an antibiotic. He simply recommended Co-Tylenol and told me to discontinue the Cytoxan until I returned for the next injection. "You need to build your white count back up," he explained.

I was discouraged and frightened. If I couldn't tolerate even the first cycle of therapy, the medicine couldn't fight the cancer.

Already the medication represented a type of security to me.

"Chemotherapy, Ron, Kris and our two little ones, my job—I just don't seem to have the strength to cope with it all, Lord. I guess I don't feel very thankful, and the Thanksgiving season is barely over."

"You shall mount up with wings as eagles. You'll run and not be weary."

"Fly, run?—I can't even drag myself off this couch and make it across the room without holding onto something."

"You shall walk and not faint."

"Oh, I forgot that sentence. That one definitely applies to me."

"Trust in me, child." My Father held me close to his bosom. His love strengthened me.

The following Monday I was strong enough to return to teach. I walked without fainting.

*　*　*

All my life I had reveled in the activity of Christmas, scurrying about for weeks preparing. Now I basked in the spirit of Christmas while lying on the couch. Understanding the importance of the Christmas tree to children, two friends popped in to clean so that our tree could be put up. I smiled at the results of their whirlwind of work. The house sparkled, and the living room was rearranged so that all Rex had to do that evening was bring our artificial tree up from the basement. The children raced to the attic to drag out boxes of ornaments and lights.

And Christmas, the season of hope, reigned in our home. I treasured the Christmas season, with its promise of joy, as much as the children did. From my couch, I saw Christmas through the eyes of a child once more. Renae and Neil made cards and decorations for the house. Kris, imitating Santa's elves, made gifts for her family and ours. And when the little ones had been put to bed and Kris was either sleeping or working on her gifts, Rex and I sat in the glow of the tree and the candles chatting with Ron or, alone, cuddling on the couch until we could pull ourselves from the tranquil scene to our bed for the night.

Acknowledging my limited strength, I pushed my shopping

plans back until vacation. Ironically, Rex and I, armed with a concise list and determination, completed in one day, the Saturday before Christmas, the shopping that usually took several months. My only other concession to the traditional Christmas bustle was the one batch of decorated sugar cookies that the children and I made the day before my second cycle of chemotherapy began. Since it was common knowledge that Christmas at the Brittons always included dozens of decorated cookies, several Sundays before Christmas we had been given a gigantic tray of cookies—delicacies from numerous friends who had each contributed two dozen from their own baking. We enjoyed the festivity of Christmas cookies without the labor.

In dread I rode to Youngstown on the 22nd for my injection. I reminded myself that I should be thankful that I would be home for this cycle; I wouldn't have to try to push myself to school each day. Still I could not dispel regret that nausea and weakness were to share our family's Christmas celebration. But throughout the cycle, as I suppressed belches and heaves, surrounded by my family's and friend's concern, I felt bathed in the joy of Christmas love. And I was struck with the awareness that physical suffering is not the worst kind of suffering a person can endure; Kris's and Ron's lives illustrated that fact.

For weeks Kris had lovingly toiled over gifts in anticipation of an idyllic day with her family. She had painted and framed an oil paint-by-number picture for her parents, decoupaged plaques, and designed brilliantly colored blocks for her smallest sister. For others, she painstakingly selected gifts. With eleven people in her immediate family, she looked like Santa as she packed her carefully wrapped presents in two large cardboard boxes.

Kris's sister was scheduled to arrive at one o'clock Christmas Eve afternoon. Dressed early, Kris paced as the minutes ticked by. Unable to be patient any longer, at three o'clock Kris called to see why her ride was late and learned that her sister wouldn't pick her up. Something had "come up."

"That's O.K." I reassured her. "We'll go past your mom's in the morning when we go to Grandma's, and we'll pick you up on the way home Christmas night."

"You can't do that. You aren't safe at my house," Kris argued illogically.

I had another idea. "Well, I'm sure Ron would be glad to take you when he comes home from work tonight."

"I'm not going." Her black eyes snapped.

I knew that there was no use arguing with her. Gently I suggested another alternative. "Why don't you just go to Grandma's with us?"

"If I can't have Christmas with my family, I won't have Christmas. Ron and I will stay home together."

Another problem, I thought. I knew Ron was afraid of what people might say if he were alone with any female. He would certainly leave if she stayed.

My stomach churned, but not from chemotherapy. "Father, what am I going to do? Please let things work out with Kris." A brainstorm struck, and I flew to the bedroom door that she had slammed shut to ask her if her brother, who lived with a family nearby, planned to go home for Christmas.

"Yeah," she mumbled.

"Why don't you call and ask him for a ride?"

After several minutes of my wheedling, Kris consented to call him, but he refused to drive her unless she bought gas. Crushed again, she slammed the receiver and hung her head dejectedly. When I understood the problem, I urged her to tell him we'd be glad to give him money for gas. Pulled by her desire to go and yet repelled by her anger, Kris debated for forty-five minutes before she finally called him back.

Her brother roared in a half-hour later.

With Kris finally on her way to her family, I sank into the bliss of our traditional Christmas Eve—the cantata and candlelight service at church, a friend's open house of candy and cookies afterward, and our return home where the children were each allowed to open one gift. Enraptured by our evening, I forgot the sorrows of the world until I noticed Ron's melancholy eyes as he watched Renae and Neil ripping paper and squealing. The curve of his lips could not hide the loneliness for his own family which seeped through his eyes. For him this happiest of seasons emphasized his great loss—his separation from his three children and wife whom he still loved. No matter how much we cared, our friendship could never compensate for the absence of Ron's family.

Christmas morning the children opened the rest of our gifts and Ron's. Ron had bought a stuffed dog for Renae's collection and an antique-styled John Deere tractor for Neil. While the children played with their toys, I prepared a turkey for Ron. I told him that I had thawed the turkey before learning that my sister-in-law planned to fix the one for the family dinner. I asked him to take it out about 12:30 and told him to help himself to the extra pies I was leaving on the counter. I couldn't stand to think of his eating a peanut-butter sandwich on Christmas.

Ron had consistently refused to spend Christmas at Mom's. "I just couldn't stand being with a family. . . . It would be a constant reminder." His more positive motive for remaining home Christmas day was to give Rex and me a special present—hanging the dry wall in the entryway that Rex had built in the summer and beginning the dry wall in the dining room we were remodeling. He broke his secrecy to get my permission to go ahead with the project. Always sensitive, Ron wanted to be certain that Rex would not be offended by his help. I had assured him that Rex and I would both be thrilled with this gift!

I spent Christmas day nibbling, napping and basking in the safety of the haven of my family's love. In the evening, we returned home to find Ron glowing with pride at accomplishing the dry-wall project. Typically he had also taken time to completely debone the turkey so that I would not have to work when I got home. As a family we sat by the tree-light enjoying the last few hours of Christmas. Ron's project had given him a sense of usefulness and an air of peace.

Our peaceful hiatus was short-lived. At eight o'clock the morning after Christmas, the phone shrilled. Kris's pleading voice directed me to pick her up on a bridge near her home as soon as I could get there. When she was warm, clean and relaxed, she told me the story of the Christmas row, which ended in her trudging through the snow to a friendly neighbor who let her sleep on the couch until morning when she walked to the local gas station to make a collect call to us. As she told me her tale, I inwardly seethed. All Kris's dreams about an ideal Christmas had been destroyed—all the work on her gifts was futile. If given the chance, I would not trade my family's acceptance and support even for perfect health.

While we were wrestling with Kris's depression over Christmas, a phone call summoned Rex and me to Children's Services to discuss her case. I made an appointment for the 29th, the day I had to return to Youngstown for the second injection of my second cycle.

The head of the agency and the caseworker's supervisor sat like presiding judges when I entered the conference room. They peered at me and inquired pointedly about my health. I brushed the issue away with "I'm just fine" and steered the conversation back to Kris. Within moments, our façades melted and we honestly hashed over the problems with Kris, her family and ours. The supervisor then asked, "How can we assist you?"

I had carefully thought out an answer to this question. "Help us guide her into further education and a career." If she didn't have definite plans by the time she was eighteen, she might drift back into her old environment and never have a productive life. We wanted the agency to shoulder some of the responsibility for Kris's future.

I left the agency relieved emotionally but drained physically. As a friend drove, I closed my eyes and leaned against the headrest, but I could not relax. My mind hummed, " 'Tis the season to be mournful." I tried to smother my depressing jingle.

That afternoon's inability to rest was typical of the three months since my surgery. At first I couldn't sleep because of my inability to find a comfortable position. Then physical discomfort was compounded by mental stress—dealing with the gossip about my condition, the uncertainties of my work schedule during my radiation treatments, the difficulties as we attempted to aid Kris's personal and academic adjustments, and our concern for Ron's and Ann's troubles. Fighting for every moment's rest, I practiced the deep-breathing techniques of natural childbirth, counting visually, singing my standard three songs and quoting Scripture. Always hours slithered by before I could fall asleep. I averted my eyes as the numbers on our digital alarm clock flipped.

I kept postponing discussing my insomnia with my doctors, for I was sure I could handle the problem myself. But now riding to the hospital, I admitted I needed help. I would ask the chemotherapist if he would prescribe a sleeping pill. I believed if I could just be knocked out, completely relaxed for several nights' rest, my body would cooperate and return to normal sleep habits. In college when I worked on a paper all night, I couldn't relax for several days. Surely overtiredness was my problem now.

My doctor did not agree with my theory, though. "Pills aren't the answer. You have to handle this problem on your own." And he lectured me sternly about the issues I must come to terms with. "I won't compound your problems by making you dependent on pills. You must depend on yourself for this victory."

Chagrined, I still admired the integrity which guided my doctor to talk to his patients rather than to placate them with pills. I meditated on his emphasis of learning to be selfish, to take time for myself. But I ignored his advice about sleeping pills and asked our neighborhood pharmacist to select an over-the-counter product that would be safe with my medication. After just several days, I found falling asleep a much easier job.

But maybe it was the doctor's talk and not the pills that made the difference because when I purchased the sleeping pills, I also accepted a new attitude. Up until then I had struggled every public moment to wear my stone mask of health. I said I was fighting for a normal life. *If I just keep doing, people will quit talking. If I maintain my normal activity, I will win back my normal life.* But after the doctor talked to me I realized that the very act of living by others' expectations was not normal; it kept me in a constant state of hyperactivity.

I vowed to sever the link between my self-esteem and my ability to do and to appear. I vowed to concentrate on my capacity to be. I acknowledged that I had to make concessions to my limited strength. It was true that my person was unaltered. I was still Janet—the same mind, the same personality, the same spirit. All those who loved *me* knew the changes in my dwelling were only surface changes—my essence was unaffected. But I had to admit and come to terms with my body's changes.

I had to evaluate each activity. Was it important to me and the family, or was it only important to maintaining the appearance of health? If it was important to me, I might choose to go to dinner with friends Friday night even though I knew I would have to sleep most of the day Saturday. But I would refuse to attend a committee meeting simply because others expected it of the healthy Janet.

I also had to accept that I had lost my ability to deal with unnecessary stress. For example, a week before Christmas when playing the organ at church I hit the chimes by mistake. I found it took several days before I could relax about that error. So now in spite of Rex's objections and my own desire to continue presurgery activities, I resigned as church organist.

I began to reshape my life around the principle that Christ's "yoke is easy." He had promised me strength for the work that he gave me. When I don't have the stamina for a job, it must be that I'm cluttering my life with nonessentials. My primary New Year's resolution for 1981 was to select carefully my priorities in spite of pressure from family and friends.

"And, Father, help me know what my priorities should be."

Life
Goes
On

I PULLED INTO A COCOON, ENCIRCLED BY OUR EXTENDED family, by my work, and by the medical routine. I tried to ignore assaults on the walls of this secure world.

The Children's Services agency's supposed help rocked our home. In a spurt of efficiency, they rescheduled an appointment for Kris with a psychologist, an appointment which was to have taken place the previous May. The psychologist assigned Kris to a vocational counselor who talked, filled out forms, determined Kris's eligibility for complete financial aid for technical training, and eventually sent her a perfunctory notice that funding for the program had been discontinued. The burden of guiding her remained with us—her surrogate parents.

My cocoon was rocked, too, by the winds of gossip. Ron's presence in our extended family fueled comments through the grapevine. "Janet and Rex have no business taking in someone else." "How can she expect to get well if she doesn't take better care of herself?" "They should let someone else worry about Ron. They aren't the only people in the church and community. Let someone else do it."

And I had to question, "Father, is caring for Ron one of the good works you have created us for?"

It seemed, as in the story of the Good Samaritan, that if there were others who could have helped, they were walking on the other side of the road ignoring the need. Our obligation to help our friend was unqualified by questions of convenience or health.

"I've promised you, child, that my burden would be light," our Father assured us, and once again he kept his promise. From Ron we received more than we gave. He brightened our home with his humor. He sat in the evenings and talked with Kris, counseling and guiding her when I could only crawl up the stairs to bed after supper. In fact, no matter how hard Ron's day had been, he refused to sit down in the evening until all my work was done and I was settled.

A morning routine developed. Rex usually left for work between five and six o'clock, and I left for school shortly before seven-thirty. Ron's job didn't begin until eight o'clock. For years on the farm, he had been working by four. Now he lay in bed until five, dressed, talked to Rex when he stumbled down the stairs, and then read or wrote letters to his three children. By the time I was dressed and downstairs, Ron was organizing a breakfast tailored to each individual. Renae's menu fluctuated with her moods. Since I conscientiously followed a high-protein diet, Ron scrambled or fried eggs for me each morning. No matter what the rest of us ate, Neil requested pancakes. Ron buttered several pieces of toast to hand to Kris as we raced for the car. With its windshield cleaned of frost and snow, the car sat, engine running, by the house. Like an efficient doorman, Ron never failed to have it ready.

Even though my concern for Kris and Ron rocked my cocoon from time to time, I cherished its safe comfort more than ever before. To this haven I dragged myself from school each day, flopped onto the couch and fell instantly asleep for an hour's nap. I turned to simple meals. For the first time in my life I began to use convenience foods—frozen chicken, frozen fish sticks, frozen french fries. Food preparation became even easier when, in January, friends bought a new microwave and sold us their used one. From that time on, I didn't argue when Ron returned home late from working on his building and insisted on reheating his own supper.

I looked forward to Wednesdays and weekends when Mom came up and did the cooking and helped organize the cleaning and washing. The children became great helpers too, cleaning and folding and putting away clothes. Renae helped cook. Neil became the official sweeper, for I did not have the stamina to push the Kirby. Rex, Mom and Kris did all the grocery shopping. To me walking the aisles seemed as impossible a feat as running a marathon. Normally an avid specials shopper and coupon clipper, I tried to ignore the strain on the budget created by the extra grocery expenses. And friends aided the family in a thousand thoughtful ways—cooking a meal, baking a pie or some cookies, cleaning a room.

My energy for dealing with people and with housework was regulated by my cycle of therapy. And just as radiation therapy had become routine, so chemotherapy settled into a familiar pattern. In fact perhaps because of the uncertainty of the future, even of reactions to that day's treatment, I, like the other chemo patients, wrapped the comforting routine around me as Linus does his blanket.

Each treatment day the dish of hard candy on the receptionist's desk confronted me with the imminent necessity of masking my metallic mouth. As I waited to speak to the receptionist, I read the notices announcing meetings of support groups with names such as Living with Cancer, I Can Cope, Make Today Count. I read warnings about Laetrile, guidelines for preparation for death, and financial suggestions from the American Cancer Society. I scanned the scribbled coloring-book pages which plastered the remaining spaces on the walls outside the receptionist's window. And silently I prayed that the "artists" —Kari, John, Becky and Eric—were little ones waiting with relatives and not pale leukemia patients.

When it was my turn, I stepped to the window. The receptionist looked into my face and smiled. "Hello, Janet. Here's your ticket." I took the slip on which the doctor would write the charges for the day and turned back to choose a chair from those that lined both sides of the hall. I scanned the faces of those around me. Here the patients were not as easy to distinguish as they had been in the radiation clinic, for there were no telltale external marks, although a few obviously wore wigs and others had wiry strands pulled into a variety of styles. As weeks passed I became increasingly grateful for Mark, my beautician, who skillfully restyled my hair as it became less healthy and thinner.

I think what struck me the most about the waiting patients was our uniqueness. Although most of the patients scheduled with me appeared to be in their early fifties or older, that was about their only common trait. Several individuals etched themselves on my memory. One sixty-year-old strawberry blonde talked of going to spend a day at the lake with her husband. "My husband wanted me to stay home and take care of myself, but I told him it was as easy to be sick on a boat in the middle of a lake as it is to be sick at home." We exchanged hints for nausea control and admitted our tendencies to nibble starchy foods to counteract the indigestion. She had me touch a lump on her clavicle as big as a baseball. The nurse called her. She returned in minutes. Once more her blood count was too low for her to tolerate a treatment. She smiled. Inwardly I mourned for her.

I was impressed by a girl, a college freshman, who had had a form of blood cancer for two years. She was feeling great and was able to go to school every day. She hoped this blood test would verify that she didn't need to go back on treatment. I hoped with her.

A handsome young man, windburned and wearing a jogging suit, leaned against the wall and shifted his weight impatiently. "Do you know that fellow?" I asked the woman next to me. "I can't believe he's a patient. He looks terrific—the picture of health."

"You should have seen him a year ago. He could barely walk.

He was thirty pounds lighter, sallow and bald. But he's no longer on treatment." This information buoyed up my hopes.

But people like the handsome jogger were always countered by others. One day I observed three attractive women. I could not distinguish which of these educated gentlewomen was the patient until one stood as her name was called. Later I described the blonde woman to my nurse and commented, "She doesn't look like a patient. Is she just here for follow-up checkups?"

In a hushed voice, the nurse answered, "She has been coming for treatments for several years. But her prognosis is not very hopeful. She works and keeps active. We all love her."

I ignored the nurses' oft-repeated advice not to build fear by comparing myself to others. Hundreds of times I was told, "Each case is unique." Yet whenever I saw the blonde, I noted her carefully styled hair, her perfectly applied, muted make-up and her placid countenance, and I smiled at her. But I could not bring myself to speak through the lump that formed in my throat for her—and for myself.

Usually I covered my sadness for fellow patients and my nervousness about the treatment by chattering incessantly to my driver.

For my examination I was ushered past the laundry bag in the hall to one of three examining rooms where the nurse and I chatted while she rapidly stabbed my finger to check my blood count. Some of the nurses just pricked the skin and caused almost no pain. Others seemed to ram the spear in so far that they had to pull it out of the fingernail on the other side. Since chemotherapy affects the bone marrow where red and white blood cells and platelets are formed, these regular blood checks assured the doctor that these blood components were maintaining acceptable levels. Once a nurse indiscreetly mentioned that radiation and chemotherapy could kill people—that the treatment could be as dangerous as the disease. I remembered how a friend's son had been cured of leukemia only to die from a hole in his lung caused by an overdose of radiation. I was thankful for the chemotherapist's cautious monitoring of my blood.

When the nurse left, I stripped from the waist up and tied the hospital gown at the back of my neck. Then I sat on the edge of the table, swinging my feet as I recorded again the stark cubicle's features. Piped-in background music played as I studied the examining table, a stool, a single straight-backed chair and a small table containing boxes of dressings, Band-Aids and glass plates for the blood smears. I avoided looking at the reflection of my concave left side in the small rectangular mirror on the wall. Many days I asked for a blanket to wrap around me as I waited. Goosebumps raised on my arms, and my teeth chattered with cold.

At last I would hear the shuffle of the doctor's feet as he paused to snatch my ticket and chart from the holder on the door. "How are you today, Mrs. Britton?" he would ask, fixing his gaze on my face and waiting for my response. Each day he carefully noted my comments. Then he thoroughly checked all over my body for lumps. He stressed repeatedly that I should call immediately, day or night, if I developed any unusual symptoms. His concern reemphasized the seriousness of the treatments.

As soon as the doctor closed the door behind him, I grabbed my clothes, threw them on and rushed to the large communal treatment room. I avoided having the injection in the windowless examining room. There I felt isolated, alone. On the other hand, the openness and noise of the communal room made me feel a part of humanity. In this room were five straight-backed chairs and four chaise longues. By each was an adjustable stand.

I wrestled with conflicting emotions as I sat in this room waiting for the results of the blood test. Expecting nausea, gas and increased weakness, part of me wished the doctor would determine that my count was too low to have the injection. Another part of me realized I needed the injection to fight the cancer. And this rational part thankfully watched as the nurse brought several syringes and rested them on the table by me. I turned my head as she tightened the tourniquet around my arm and warned, "Just a little pinch now." First she drew my blood and then she eased in the medication, using the same site to save my veins from collapse. After several treatments, the nurses had more difficulty finding a vein. They asked me to pump my arm, and they slapped

LIFE GOES ON ————————————————————————————173

it rapidly to raise one to the surface. Hearing other patients talk, I feared the day that the needle would have to be stuck in my hand or even in my elbow. I cherished the last faithful vein on the inside of my arm, obsessed with its not failing me.

Sometimes when I turned my head to avoid seeing my injection, I would catch a glimpse of a needle piercing someone's arm. Quickly I'd clamp my eyes shut and block the scene from my memory. But although I never watched the liquid infusing my vein, I could always easily judge its progress. The creeping metallic secretion under my tongue accompanied the sensation of the medicine rushing into my vein.

The nurses insisted that I remain in the communal room until the clamminess and the first wave of nausea passed. I declined their offers of injections for nausea (although I accepted the prescription for suppositories and pills) because I prefer nausea to needles.

I always wanted to escape "cancer's confines" immediately, but bureaucracy mandated that patients settle bills in the insurance office after every injection. The paperwork could not be completed before the injection because the doctor often readjusted dosage at each visit. I resented the delay. Barely civil, I answered the questions, filled out the papers and wobbled to the car.

By the time we reached the city limits, I was burping frequently while munching on the potato chips and sipping the cola that I hoarded for the trip home. I learned quickly that immediately after a treatment I craved salt and anything with tomato sauce. The children, who always greeted me at the door by asking "Did they get those bad cells, Mom?" looked forward to my treatments because we developed the tradition of ordering pizza, cola and chips for supper.

*   *   *

A young medical student who interviewed me as part of a study on chemotherapy-related nausea told me that Compazine suppositories and pills are not adequate for many people. THC, a derivative of marijuana, helps some, but not all. Her thesis was that hypnosis might be most effective, especially for patients who become nauseated and begin vomiting even before the actual injection. Because of my own escalating dread of entering the department of oncology and hematology, I could understand why some patients begin vomiting in anticipation of the chemical assault on the digestive tract. Waiting for the reactions that varied in severity from treatment to treatment was excruciating.

Perhaps because we had no control over our physical responses to treatment, most of us seized control over aspects of the treatment itself. Just as I clung past all reason to my favorite vein, so one woman refused to walk through the annex entry. She traveled a long circuitous route from the emergency room entrance to the back hall of the oncology department. Insisting that an odor by the door suffocated her, she would not pass the sign labeling her a cancer patient. Periodically when she feared that the odor permeated the whole department, her favorite nurse would arrange to meet her in the emergency room to administer treatments until the odor subsided and again she could force herself to sneak in the back way.

Linked to our need for control was our adopting favorite nurses. One gained the title of "my nurse" because "I don't get sick when she gives me the injection." Another was chosen because "she looks just like my youngest granddaughter." Mine acquired her favored status because she was the first one I didn't have to ask not to say "just a little pinch now," "we're almost through" or "just a little longer." Instinctively she talked only of her fiancé, my work and graduate classes, our families and hairdos.

Most of us developed a ritualistic menu to help us cope with the nausea. My choice of pizza, potato chips and cola was just one example. One elderly woman spent her time in the waiting room preaching that eating macaroni and cheese before each treatment is the sure antidote for nausea and vomiting. Another patient cried the merits of eating french bread immediately after treatments. Still another insisted peppermint candy is the answer. To each of us the staff answered sincerely, "If it works for you, it's true."

Each oncology nurse seemingly wore antennae designed to

sense every innuendo, heed every passing remark that would add to her storehouse of understanding. The nurses' attitudes reflected their belief in the impact of psychological factors on chemo's effectiveness. As a unit they encouraged us to be happy and avoid stress. No one even subtly scoffed at our superstitious adherence to patterns. The staff saw our self-imposed routines as the garments we clothed ourselves in to protect us from exposure to fear and frustration.

But the oncology staff's respect for individual choice was not typical of the general public. People observing my weakness offered me hundreds of "helpful" suggestions. I was offered vitamin capsules, vegetable juices, new diets, addresses of miracle doctors and articles on "the latest approach to the treatment of cancer." I was urged to consider the nontoxic approach of a clinic in the Bahamas. I listened. I thanked people for their concern. But having made the decision, I continued my treatments, although I once asked Rex, "Don't you think a daily dosage of D-Con Rat Killer would be cheaper and less trouble than my chemotherapy?" He didn't smile.

But he did smile at my declaration of a moratorium on the "fat and bald" jokes I made about him. Struggling not to gain too much weight from the therapy and continually rearranging my own thinning strawlike hair, I thought I was not one to be casting stones. The pathetic humor of my chemo-ridden body struck me one day as Rex helped me from the tub where the drain held a handful of my hair and the bathroom floor held my breast. "At least my teeth aren't in a jar on the sink yet," I consoled myself.

My weakness, nausea, dizziness, hair loss and mouth sores were typical effects of chemotherapy. But one of my chronic irritations shows how differently each individual reacts to chemicals. Some people have no side effects. Others, like me, develop symptoms that are not usually linked to a drug. My eyelids swelled and light bothered me. I squinted continually and resorted to wearing dark glasses.

*   *   *

Of all my symptoms, though, the most widely discussed was

the breathing problem that began during the last weeks of radiation and continued for months. One of the first people to comment on my labored breathing was the school secretary. One day toward the end of my radiation therapy, I trotted into the office to hand her a form. She stared at me and asked, "Janet, what on earth have you been doing?"

"I haven't been doing anything unusual. Why?"

"You sound as if you've just run a mile, puffing like that. What does your doctor say about your breathing?"

"I don't know. I never mentioned it. I assume it's just a side effect of the radiation. My lungs are probably dried out like my skin is. I look like a lizard."

But my breathing problem did not improve when radiation ended. Increasingly, the simplest exercise—standing, walking— left me winded. I wheezed like a steam engine and gasped between phrases in conversation. I could not sing or hum a line without dissolving into paroxysms of coughing. I had to avoid the teachers' lunchroom because the cigarette smoke started me choking almost nonstop for several hours. Even strangers began to joke about my "smoker's cough."

Trying to control my dry hacking, I talked softly so as not to expel too much air and irritate my throat. At night I lay still, face down, holding my breath to suppress coughs. My heart beat wildly through the thin layer of skin that covered the left side of my chest. The bed shook as I pressed my arms firmly across my rib cage to counteract the coughing reflex. I began to spend my night propped with pillows in our living room recliner.

I lived with a Hall's cough drop tucked in my mouth. Since I preferred the cherry-flavored ones, my tongue had an almost permanent red stain. Continually I brushed my mouth to remove the red slime. I sampled every cough medicine on the market that did not contain the lethargy-inducing codeine. In desperation I borrowed a partially filled flask from a friend so that I could mix the cough medicine the pediatrician had prescribed for one of Renae's coughs—honey, lemon and vodka.

My labored breathing caused my family growing concern. Mom acted on her concern. One Wednesday she informed me,

"I made an appointment with Dr. Mann for next Monday. He's an excellent diagnostician, very straightforward, and he spends a lot of time with each patient. I'm sure you'll like him."

But I told her she might as well cancel the appointment. I refused to go.

"Just think about it," she cajoled me. "Do it for me if for no other reason. I'd feel so much better if you'd see him."

"I'm sick of wasting half my life sitting in doctors' waiting rooms," I retorted.

"Just one more time, dear. Just so I won't worry so much." Her brown eyes penetrated my defenses. Guilt trickled through the cracks of my stubbornness. I could not subject my mother to more worry. Monday, like a reluctant child obeying her mother, I drove from school to the doctor's office.

My jaw clamped tightly when I stomped through the doors of the clinic. What a waste of time, I thought.

The doctor's nurse filled out a questionnaire. "Regular medications?" she asked.

"I'm on chemotherapy," I said.

The nurse shifted her eyes slightly. I gazed at her intently, following carefully my role as the "cancer patient who can cope!"

The interview ended with her order, "Step behind the screen, remove your clothes, put on this gown, and tie it in the back."

"Thank you, but I won't be needing that," I responded evenly. "I just came for consultation."

"But the doctor will need to examine you."

"I had an examination just last week." I did not flinch.

Slightly flustered, the nurse stammered, "Well, well . . . the doctor will be with you soon."

I graded the papers I had brought into the examining room with me. As I sat, I mentally argued, "Why should I put on a gown? Does he need to see the scar to understand that I have no breast? Why does the patient have to be undressed to carry on a conversation? Why do medical people think patients are mindless lambs?" I grew increasingly agitated at the wait.

My ramblings were interrupted by a tall, fortyish man who confidently strode through the door, smiling and nodding at me as he pushed the curtain back. He halted abruptly. Bewildered, he gazed at the vacant examining table.

Reading his confusion, I explained, "I'm the patient."

"Oh?"

"My cough has made everyone say I need a medical doctor, so I came to see you."

He checked my questionnaire, regained his composure and asked me about my medical history since August. "I wouldn't prescribe anything, even for a cold, without verifying the exact protocol of your chemotherapy," he said. "Any medication would have to be approved by your chemotherapist."

"That's what I thought. But the staff at Youngstown says I need to have a medical doctor check my cough."

The typical runaround, I thought. But Mom was right. This doctor took time with his patient. He tilted back on his chair, chewed his pencil and puckered his brow. "To me your dry cough sounds exactly like a radiation cough. The drying-out process of radiation lasts months. Even though you haven't had treatments for quite some time, I'm quite sure that cough is the result of the therapy."

He warmed to the topic. "In my experience, I have found cancer a strange disease. In one case I remember, the bone was affected before the lump in the breast was large enough to detect. Yet another woman ignored a lump for twelve years. By the time we saw her, the breast was seriously macerated, yet there was no metastasis to the bones or even to the lymph nodes. We just don't have the answers about cancer's effects."

I enjoyed our conversation. I was beginning to understand why Mom's friends liked the man. As our chat concluded, he said, "If you'd like to make another appointment, I'd like to listen to your lungs to verify that the cough is from radiation."

"Well, would you like to examine me now?" I asked, confused.

"I thought you didn't want to undress for some reason."

"No," I laughed. "I don't want to undress for no reason. If there is a purpose, I don't object to an exam."

"Then please step behind the curtain. I'll be right with you. You just need to disrobe from your waist up."

Again the absurdity of medical conventions hit me. I stepped modestly behind a curtain and put on a gown so that within moments he could open the curtain and lift the gown.

*　　*　　*

Kris refused to go to school on Friday, the last day of February. I had been absent the previous Wednesday; weak from an injection, I had propped myself on the couch all day, reading a book for my graduate study and listening as Ron discussed his fears that Ann might begin divorce proceedings. Thursday I had managed to drag both Kris and myself to school. But Friday morning, too weak to force a confrontation, I left her curled peacefully under her blankets.

At 3:45 I opened the laundry room door. It had been a long day.

"I have a whole list of phone messages for you," Kris announced before I had a chance to drag myself into the kitchen. "Ann called. She's in town and will be here in about fifteen minutes. Ron called several times, and he said he'd call back."

I dropped my books on the counter and reached for the teakettle. Kris plopped onto a kitchen chair and hesitantly continued, "I want to apologize for not going to school again. Ron called me this morning from work just to try to explain how difficult it is for you as a teacher to be legally responsible for me and have me skipping school. I guess I never thought about the trouble I cause you."

Before I drained the last gulp of my tea, Ann arrived. Tall and lithe, her hair attractively streaked, she looked great. Kris disappeared to give us privacy. We clung to each other for several minutes. Almost a year had passed since we had seen each other in person. She asked about my health. I asked about her graduate courses and what had prompted her to make the nine-hour drive without any notice.

"I just had a free day and decided to come up to get some old notes for a nutrition class paper. I guess I wanted to see home again. But it has turned out to be a horrible afternoon. The tenant at the farm said he couldn't let me in the house because the place is not legally ours; it belongs to Ron's dad and he left orders to keep me out."

She had called Ron to defend her and Ron had left work to meet her at the farm. Ron told the tenant that he would personally take responsibility for Ann's entering so that any problem would be between Ron and his dad. The tenant still would not permit Ann in the house, although he partially relented, saying Ron could get what Ann needed. Finally conceding defeat, Ron asked Ann to describe the papers she wanted and explain their location.

"I just refused. We lived in that house for thirteen years. We put our lives into that farm while all Ron's folks did was interfere in our home." Her voice rose and her face flushed. She stopped herself, took a deep breath and continued more calmly. "I couldn't explain which papers I wanted anyway."

After the fiasco at the farmhouse, Ron had given her a tour of his building and showed his plans to her. "I kept telling him how nice it was going to be but that we aren't coming back. I don't think he wants to accept that." She changed the topic back to children and to college courses.

In the middle of our conversation, the phone rang. Ron's voice boomed over the wires. "Try to talk to Ann. She's really upset. I'm worried that . . ."

I cut him short so that Ann would not be inhibited by knowing that the call was from Ron. "I understand. Yes, I'll talk to you later. Bye."

In spite of my caution, Ann stayed only a few more minutes before she stood and said that she needed to begin her long return trip to Virginia.

While I was browning the hamburger for chili, Ron came home from work. He told Rex that his boss was upset with him for leaving that afternoon. "He threatened to fire me, but I don't think he meant it," he said, brooding. He stared into space for a few minutes and then turned on his heels and darted to the basement to change into heavier clothes so he could work on his house in the February cold.

As I cooked, I hollered down the stairs, trying to draw him into a conversation. I tried to convince him that Ann was no longer upset. He disagreed. "She said she'd never set foot in Andover again."

I tried to convince him otherwise. "She may have said that to you, but she talked to me about the kids coming for the summer. She talked about seeing me soon. You know she was just upset. Sometimes we say things we don't mean when we're uptight. She was just fine by the time she left."

Ron didn't answer me. I chatted on, attempting to soothe his pain.

I tried to detain him by inviting him to wait just a few more minutes to eat with us. But bundled in heavy work clothes, Ron rushed up the steps seemingly driven by a silent force. I felt compelled to keep him from bolting away. I reached out and touched his arm. He halted, but he did not look at me. "You know we love you, Ron. You know how much you mean to all of us. Things will work out."

He stood like a statue. Without responding, he threw open the door, leaped into his pickup and rattled out the driveway.

I drifted into the living room and perched on the arm of Rex's chair. We debated whether we should follow him. We wanted to do the right thing. Rex hesitated. "You know how proud he is."

Yes, I mused. Ron obviously wanted to be alone. But I wasn't positive we should let him go off by himself. "He's so upset. He might just go wreck the house instead of building it. I've never seen him so depressed."

"It might be the best thing if he did. Just take out his frustrations on his pipe dream." Rex stroked his chin and sighed. "But whatever he does, he needs to be by himself to get himself together. You know how he hates anyone to see him lose control."

The evening passed. I crawled into bed the minute our friends, who had dropped by for the evening, left. I was not surprised that Ron wasn't home. He often worked late on weekends.

When we woke the next morning, though, Ron still wasn't home. Before Rex went to play basketball at 8:30, he checked to make sure that Ron's truck was at his building. It was. Obviously Ron had worked late and slept there. Rex went on with the church team.

A friend came about ten o'clock and took Renae and Neil for

an outing. I painted woodwork, preparing the house for Kris's graduation open house.

When Rex returned for lunch, his first question was, "Has Ron been back?"

"No."

I flipped a hamburger. Nothing more was said for several minutes. I pressed the issue. "You know you have to go talk to him, honey."

Neither of us voiced our gnawing belief that Ron surely had wrecked the house that he had slaved over for three months. Weeks of frustration had wound up his emotions like a time bomb set for an unspecified hour. Last night that hour had come.

Rex was hesitant. "I don't know if I'll be able to handle him. I don't know if I'll find the right thing to say."

"You're his friend. He knows that. Anything you say out of love will be fine. If you want, though, I'll call Gary. Maybe he'd go with you. The two of you could just casually drop in on the pretense of helping him this afternoon." (Genny and her husband, Gary, had been friends of Ann and Ron, too, for many years.)

Rex left. Kris and I patched the wallpaper around the slightly smaller new window that Rex had installed in Neil's room. Giggling and talking, we pasted the last piece of the car print and were gathering brushes to wash when a car slid to a halt in our driveway. I looked out the window. It was Gary and Genny.

My stomach dropped. Where was Rex? Why had Gary gone back to his house for Genny? I knew something had to be wrong.

I rushed downstairs to open the laundry room door. Gary spoke. "Ron hanged himself." His words echoed in my brain like a foreign phrase. Painfully, I translated those syllables into a horrible unreality. The sequence of events blurred. I moved in slow motion. I struggled to wake from the nightmare.

Friends came to the house, sat silently, put an arm around each of us, left. Kris floated by. I reached out to touch her. She smiled. I was comforted by the fuzzy awareness that she is a survivor—a master of the endurance of pain. The children returned. How does one explain death to a child? An accident or an illness is difficult but understandable, for we had taught them that eventually God takes people who love him to live with him in heaven. But God didn't choose this; Ron himself chose death. He chose to inflict pain on himself and on the people who love him.

The children sat on our bed for a family conference—a conference that was going to be much more devastating than the one before my surgery. The children had already heard that Ron was dead. Now we had to answer the question "What happened?" Rex was the spokesman. "You know Ron was very unhappy without Ann and the kids." He stopped—no words were appropriate. "Sometimes when we get depressed we won't let the people who love us, even God, help us." He stopped again. He pulled Renae and Neil tightly against his chest and gazed over their blond heads. His eyes beseeched me to give him the words.

Neil pulled back, cocked his head and with a furrowed forehead innocently said, "He didn't commit suicide, did he?"

Rex buried his face on Neil's chest. "How do you understand so easily when I can't?" Sobs rent his body. The four of us encircled each other's shoulders. But we could not reach each other's deep wounds.

Kris scampered up the stairs holding her pillow. "I'm going to sleep upstairs tonight." She didn't want to be alone.

The next morning Rex met with the coroner to give him Ron's suicide note and to describe the discovery of Ron's body. Ann and the children arrived from Virginia. Ron's parents and his few relatives drove in from out of town.

Sunday Rex helped Ann make funeral arrangements—service times, favorite music, a cemetery plot, a marker. We prepared the children for the funeral ceremony. We attended church services. I taught an adult Sunday-school class. "Pray for the Bonner family," I said. And silently added, "for the Britton family too."

During the day Rex was a rock—for our children, for Ron's children, for his chosen sister, Ann. At night he shook in grief over the loss of his friend, over his own inability to understand or prevent Ron's act of despair. Repeatedly he fixed his attention on space and sighed. "No one can ever tell me that that was the

coward's way out; no one could say that if they had seen him."
Never a word more about any of the images that had seared themselves on his brain.

"I was closer to him than to my natural family. He was like a
brother."

He nursed the emotional wounds of Ron's family as if they
were his own.

"Do you think it would bother the children if Ron was buried
next door?" Rex asked. A small country cemetery borders our
farm to the north.

"Ask them."

Our children were delighted at the thought. "If they bury Ron
in the cemetery next to us, we can watch him for Susan and Elizabeth and Rob." I observed their optimistic planning, fearing that
I would not accept the proximity of his grave as easily as the
children. The children's resilience once more astounded me. Then
Rex added, "I reserved the lots next to Ron. I told the funeral
director that I'd like to check your opinion first."

I hesitated. I realized that I was not "well-adjusted" enough
to relish buying our cemetery plots. Not now at least.

Rex explained his views. "We have spent so much time together. I thought we might as well stay together to the end."

I gave in. Rex had stronger feelings for buying the lots than I
had against buying them.

The blurred events of that week are interspersed within a
montage of mental pictures of the children. One image is of Neil
and Susie sitting on the top bunk. Susie closes the door when
she sees me. "We'd like to talk private. We're talking about my
daddy." The camera of my mind clicks. Renae and Elizabeth
arranging the "prettiest" flowers on Ron's grave. Click. Neil
huddled in a fetal position under the blankets of Ron's "bed"—
the sleeping bag arranged on the foam mattress. Neil whimpers
as he dreams. Click. The three girls holding imaginary micro-
phones, singing with a Kenny Rogers album: "Good friend. Why
did you have to go? Just when I was getting to know you. . . ."
Click. A tear slips down my cheek. My tears flood out the images.

Wednesday after the funeral I helped Ann supervise the men

from the church as they loaded the U-Haul truck at the farm. I continued on cruise control as my mind dwelt on this most final type of death—the death of all hope of ever recapturing the past, the end of what we'd shared as families. No more anniversary dinners. No more evening picnics at the lake. No more barbecues after a day of planting. No more watermelons or ice cream after haying. No "clean-the-refrigerator" pizzas on winter evenings. No sharing of trips to the hospital, babysitting or tutoring each other's children.

No listening to the Bonner and Britton children as they laugh on the swing set or squeal down the slide or giggle in the play-house over the workshop or peel rubber with bike tires in the lane. No watching them carry a snake from the creek or sew a doll dress or assemble a puzzle. Never again would they feed a new-born calf with a bottle for the payment of a piece of Ron's hard candy from the bag in the milk house.

From this time on, toll calls would be the tenuous link between our families. We could have reunions. But we could never re-capture the life we'd lost. This ripping apart of our enmeshed lives was more final than death itself—and more difficult to accept.

*   *   *

The U-Haul truck, driven by Ann's Virginia friends, left. But the freshly dug grave in the small cemetery past our apple trees remained. The vacuum in our hearts remained with it.

The children frequently referred to this painful void. They took turns starting and warming the car "just like Ron always did." Renae slept with the stuffed dog that "Ron bought me for Christ-mas." "If Ron were here, he'd fix my pancakes" became Neil's morning litany.

And inevitably they asked, "Why? Ron read his Bible. Why didn't he pray and let God help him?"

"Sometimes we're too stubborn to ask for help. Remember when I try to help you and you say you want to do it yourself? Sometimes even adults are like that with God."

They studied the cold facts of *suicide*. Renae discussed some of her research into this topic with me.

"Jennifer said Ron choked himself. That isn't true, is it?"

"Yes, it's true."

"How could he do that?"

"With a rope."

"That's terrible."

"Yes, it is. He was very upset to do that. He wouldn't let anyone help him with his problems." (I heard Jesus mourn, "How often I longed to protect him, as a hen gathers her chicks under her wings, but Ron was not willing.")

"I don't want to think about it." Renae set her jaw.

I held her. "Then don't, honey. Think of how much fun you had when you helped him in the hayfield and in the barn feeding the calves. Think of how he loved peanut dogs and how he held Susan and Elizabeth. Think of how the cats and Barney [his German Shepherd] followed him all over the farm. Think of how he laughed. Think of those things when you think of our friend Ron."

I kissed her. She ran up the stairs, smiling.

I prayed, "Teach me how to follow my own advice."

*   *   *

For weeks as I sat at the clinic, I debated why those with only a few years left would subject themselves to the debilitation of chemotherapy. Cynically I asked Mom, "How can the researchers count some of these people as dying of cancer?" I motioned to an elderly man barely able to shuffle himself to the receptionist's desk. "Would you count him?" I whispered. I nodded to the woman, probably in her eighties, who slumped in a wheelchair. "What about her?"

"They are also individuals."

"But they would die soon anyway—just of old age."

"A moment of life is precious at any age."

The disparity of people's attitudes toward life haunted me. In the face of these elderly fighters for life, how could I accept my friend's disregard for his? I could not comprehend that Ron had willingly thrown away his life while I, and thousands of people like me, struggled madly for each day of useful life.

"Father, you don't know how I grieve for him. How can I accept the suicide of such a close friend?"

"Lean on me."

"I know. But I loved Ron so! Our family was so involved with him!"

"I know. For three years my Son and his disciples were so involved with their friend. I wanted to help but he hanged himself in a fit of depression. I grieved for him. I loved him so."

"I guess you do understand. But how can I cope?"

"Follow Paul's example when he said, 'One thing I do: forgetting what is behind and straining toward what is ahead, I press on toward the goal to win the prize for which God has called me.' "

"All right, Father. I will press on." To cope with Ron's suicide, I focused my energy on preparing for Kris's graduation. Although I couldn't handle open-ended philosophical questions about suicide, I could deal with the practical problems of redecorating for Kris's open house and filling out financial-aid forms for her further education. Our family wrapped itself up with Kris to compensate for Ron. We concentrated on the living, reminding ourselves that it was too late to help the dead. With her friends and other faculty members, we tried to convince her that her future was promising. But Kris was beginning to pull back in fear. She repeated her family's belief that "none of us will ever amount to anything," and she feared that this assessment was accurate. I desperately wanted to make Kris believe she is "somebody"—somebody very important.

Helping the children understand. Comforting my husband at the death of his best friend. Coping with my own grief. Helping Ron's family avoid the "what ifs." Facing Kris's fears of the future. Remodeling the house in time for Kris's open house. These were the immediate challenges of my life. Weak and nauseated, I forced myself up and moving each day to school where I developed a writing lab, tutored and taught.

I stayed out of the discussions that one person from the high-school English department was going to be transferred to the junior high school. For several years the two teachers with the least seniority in our department of five had been shuffled about. The matter did not involve me until one day in April when the superintendent summoned me to his office. Since I was the department head, I assumed he wanted to discuss a curriculum matter. I was unprepared for his opening statement. "We are planning to move you to the junior-high position."

Shocked, I sat mute for several minutes. Finally I collected my wits to argue that such a move would adversely affect the writing program I was developing. Ignoring my points, he continued, unctuous and flattering. "With your creativity and dedication, you will be the perfect person to improve the junior-high program. I'm sure you'll leap to this challenge."

Leaving the office, I staggered into the hall and bumped into a colleague. "Do you know what the administration is doing to me?" I blurted out.

"Yes, I've heard them talking."

I poured out my frustrations. The task of developing and implementing a new program for immature students while I was on chemotherapy seemed impossible. And I had established a reputation with the high-school students. They treated me with great consideration. In junior high, though, I'd have to cover my weakness while building a new reputation with this notoriously difficult-to-handle age group.

"What could be the reason for moving me?" I hung my head in discouragement. "Aren't the administrators interested in maintaining the writing emphasis in the high school? You would think they'd be proud that two of the programs pioneered by me were presented at a NCTE meeting."

My friend paused only a moment before answering. "To be crude—I think the administration believes you won't be teaching much longer and the disruption in the program will occur eventually anyway . . ." He shifted his weight from side to side. "Ah . . . since you probably won't live that much longer anyway."

That evening I relayed the conversations to Rex. His eyes narrowed and his jaw set. "Fight them," he spat.

"I'm too tired to fight. It's bad enough to expend twice as much energy as before to prove I can do the same job."

But Rex kept pushing me. "You know you can fight the transfer on the grounds of discrimination. The Civil Liberties Union would support you. You have evidence of the administration's attitude toward cancer. And in former years the two English teachers under you were always shuffled. Tell me what has changed except your health."

I knew Rex was right. Even more simply, I could let the teacher's association fight for me. But I could not tolerate the effort of such a fight. After deliberation, I decided to make a simple appeal in writing to the board of education. I would base my appeal on two things: the decision's effect on the curriculum and my reputation as a dedicated teacher. And then I'd abide by their decision.

Carefully, I composed a letter which reviewed the developments in the English curriculum and the board's past support of these programs. As I addressed the letter, I felt as if my job had become a foreign camp; I was surrounded by enemies.

"Child, I take care of you when you enter the clinics that you associate with the valley of the shadow of death."

"In other words, Father, you want to prepare a table before me in the presence of these enemies?"

"Of course."

"But this is a real mess. You just don't change the minds of these men once they've taken a position. It'd take a miracle to settle this!"

God smiled. I grinned foolishly and acknowledged, "I keep forgetting who I'm talking to. I know, 'Surely goodness and mercy shall follow me all the days of my life.' "

"Yes, you're learning, child. Now I can take over."

The board swiftly resolved the problem. Several days later the English teacher with least seniority was called into the superintendent's office and told she would be moved to the junior-high position. My transfer was never mentioned again.

Ron—Kris—my teaching position. During this time of strain, my physical condition deteriorated. Locomotion became increasingly difficult, for I frequently lost my equilibrium. I staggered on flat ground, pulled myself upstairs with both hands and rested on each landing, puffing. Clutching the wall as inconspicuously as possible, I groped my way down the hall to my classroom each day. I moved slowly and cautiously, keeping my head erect and fixing my eyes straight ahead to avoid any sudden movements.

Several times, involved in my teaching, I forgot my caution and almost had a disaster. For example, one day as I worked my way down the aisle answering questions, a student behind me spoke up. I rose and turned at the same time. Instantly I found myself lying over a desk, staring at the auburn hair of a macho eighteen-year-old male student. I attempted to cover my embarrassment with a tacky joke. "I'm not throwing myself at you, honestly." My students laughed with me. I shuffled to my chair for the rest of the period. Such incidents forced me to revise my classroom management by encouraging students to come to me. The desk that had been used only sporadically for nine years now received constant use. Student learning didn't seem hampered by this alteration. Students sensed that I still encouraged their questions and without hesitation they came for help.

During this time, I understood my grandmother's anger at her body's refusal to keep up the pace she wanted. I fumed at my body's refusal to move as I directed it, at its tendency to balk like a willful child. Grandma saw this connection too. One day as I walked to the house with her, holding her arm as always, she quipped, "I think this is an example of the blind leading the blind."

Dr. Bhatti, observing my dizziness, said that most likely my mobility problems, though uncommon, were related to the chemicals—probably the 5-FU. But when I remained dizzy after decreased dosage, he scheduled me for a CAT scan to rule out a brain tumor. Although I viewed the chance of having a brain tumor as remote, the doctor had originally told me that the cancer's next stage would be the bone, usually in the thoracic area, or the brain. I dreaded that possibility. The idea of losing control of mobility, speech and other functions was terrifying.

"Who of you by worrying can add a single hour to his life?"

"Yes, I hear you, Father."

"Do not let your heart be troubled."

The iodine dye was injected. I was slid into the tunnel machine and lay still as minutes tiptoed by. I staggered to the car. In a few days, I received the results. The scan was negative. My equilibrium problems were from a chemical reaction.

* * *

The major remodeling projects were completed just two days before Kris's open house; our friends joined us for a joyous celebration of her accomplishment in graduating. I finished typing the final fifty-page paper for a graduate school independent study and then concluded the school year at work—storing materials for the summer, filling out end-of-year reports, recording yearly grades. On the last day of school I rushed to enroll in a class at Kent State University. The professor said I would not have to attend this class if I would write a lengthy critique of the textbook. On the basis of this paper and the work from a previous class, he would give me a letter grade for a course which would be accepted by Youngstown State.

For three weeks after summer vacation began, while reading for and writing my critique, I lay on the beach every sunny day and watched the children splash and build sand castles. They frequently ran back to instruct me to watch their antics. On dismal days the children read and played games. I moved from the recliner to the couch and back again.

The first week of July I began a two-week writing workshop which was immediately followed by a five-week course in American fiction, my last course for my master's degree. All my energy trickled into my education. I took pride in the fact that my mind was unaffected by cancer. Though I had limited physical stamina, I had enough strength to study and to read.

For the first time I understood the driving force of mountain climbers. Formerly their goal of reaching a given altitude seemed ridiculous to me. After all, there was no reward for mankind or personal profit in climbing a mountain. In the same way, runners who devote their lives to beating a clicking clock seemed foolish. What did these things matter? But now my education was my own obsession. The more people said to relax and finish school later, the more I was determined to prove I could finish now. Sometimes I felt like the man on "That's Incredible" who played tug of war with the Goodyear blimp. The odds were seemingly insurmountable; victory was of insignificant value. Yet he, like me, was compelled to strain.

Each treatment day I was excused from class after submitting a paper that I had done as a take-home exam. The day after treatments, the children fixed breakfast and rode bikes while I lay in bed until almost noon. Then I'd drive the few miles to the beach and nap while the children played on the shore.

While I attended college and juggled my treatments, my sister and mother helped finish the work with Kris. Kris's future looked promising. I was optimistic that our family's investment in love would yield a new life for her. For one individual the cycle of despair would be broken. Generations would be positively influenced, saved from futility, abuse, emotional crippling.

Then a few fluffy cirrus clouds began to form. After completing all the papers for scholarships and grants so that she could attend computer school in the fall, Kris decided that she preferred working for at least a year. Bonnie and Mom knew the urgency of helping Kris establish some permanence. Bonnie drove Kris to numerous places to apply for work, and finally my aunt helped get her a job in a nursing home. (I thought that perhaps this job would lead to a renewed interest in becoming a practical nurse or a medical technician.) To save gas Kris moved to my mother's home which was only two miles from the nursing home. We encouraged Kris to buy a used car so that she would have independence. We helped her get title and plates.

And then the nimbus and cumulus clouds rolled in. Proudly she drove the car to her hometown. Word reached her former boyfriend. "Kris has a good job and she got her own car." He called her at our house where she was visiting. "I'm not going to go running if he didn't care enough to see me for over a year," she said as she rushed out the door to start the car that would drive her to him.

I sat discouraged, fearing this might be the first step to her return to her old life. Within days I learned that my fear was justified.

We celebrated the granting of my master's degree. I watched my tassle swinging from our car's mirror. It had been difficult, but I had reached that career goal. Yet if I'd had my choice, I would have chosen failure in academics rather than failure in our goal of helping Ron and Kris.

Kris said she had just gone to see her old boyfriend out of curiosity. She would never get involved with him again. This was the first of a series of statements telling what she'd never do just days or moments before she did that very thing. "I'll never miss work for him," Kris said days before her cycle of tardiness and absence from work began. "I'd never let him drive my car." (The boyfriend had repeatedly lost his license for driving under the influence of alcohol or other drugs.) This she said a month before he wrecked her car for the first time. "I'll never let him boss me around again," she said shortly before she visited me with a black eye, battered ribs and fingerprint bruise marks on her biceps.

I began to panic. Just as Ron committed suicide, so Kris was throwing her life away emotionally. I tried to understand her inability to live in the new world. She said she was used to her old ways. Maybe she had experienced too much pain in the past to risk hope. I remembered how I am frozen by fear at the sight of a snake. Perhaps fear makes Kris unable to move into productivity.

But I prayed for God to make her change her mind.

He answered, "You cannot make her decision for her. I won't make her decision. I have given her free will, not made her a puppet. We both must continue to love her. And wait—"

"But, Father, she might never come back."

"I know that," he sighed.

"But, Father, it's so painful to have to stand by and do nothing."

"I remember the rich young ruler."

"I don't understand."

"He went away sorrowfully—into a life that he was used to."

"Why didn't you stop him?" I argued. "Why don't you stop Kris?"

And he repeated, "I can only love them. And watch them go if they choose that."

"How can you stand to do that?"

"I tend my other sheep. And wait. You must do the same."

I remained quiet a few moments. Then I asked, "Did he ever come back—the rich young ruler, I mean?"

God smiled sadly. "That is not your concern, child," he told me gently. "You must do the works I give you. I am the tender of the harvest."

*   *   *

When I was a freshman in college, my roommate and I made a calendar of days until vacation. Each evening we tore the sheet off and threw it into the wastebasket. Once my roommate commented, "There are our lives lying in that wastebasket." I vowed I would never make the error of postponing my life again.

In September when I returned to school and to my thermometer of health, the stairs to my second-floor classroom, I forgot that old vow and began impatiently counting the time until I would be off injections. I hoped for the day that I could once more skip up the stairs two at a time as I had for years. I prayed for even just one month to feel normal. I lived in a type of suspended animation. "If I can just make it to November. If the doctor will just discontinue the medication . . ."

The old discomfort plagued me and I could not sleep. I propped my arm over my head to promote drainage of the lymph system in my left arm. I tried to disregard my body and drag through my activities. I fulfilled my duties by rote. My body forged on. My mind stagnated. My arm and shoulder ached like a bad tooth. I kept going. "Just one more month," I thought. "Then I will feel better."

At last I could not ignore the lumps spreading on my underarm. I called the doctor and he prescribed an antibiotic, but the lumps did not disappear. "I don't like your lumps and bumps," he said on the day of my last scheduled chemotherapy treatment.

The nagging fear that chemotherapy might have to continue

destroyed the elation I had anticipated at this final injection. I felt like I had the postpartum blues. A major lesson from my father's illness haunted me—cancer is never really over!

The chemotherapist sent me back to my surgeon who scheduled me for outpatient surgery to lance and biopsy the lumps. "I'm sure they are benign." His statement echoed his identical statement in August the year before. Rationally I knew this was an entirely different case, but emotionally I could not shake the nagging doubt.

I tried to appear nonchalant as I registered and undressed, was medicated and taken to the holding area outside the operating room. Five of us waited. Only inches separated us. Yet over the room hung the silence of dumb beasts herded into stalls in the slaughterhouse. I remembered previously feeling like a pagan sacrifice.

In defiance I sat up Indian-style and observed the controlled flurry of the operating room staff. Almost immediately a nurse dashed to my side and, gasping, scolded me. "You can't sit up here!"

Prepared for such an order, I declared, "Since I got cancer, I've learned that the hospital's rules aren't chiseled in stone. Just give me a release to sign."

She was not impressed with my reasoning. "I have cancer too, and I follow the rules."

Chagrined, I hesitated. Her voice changed and she cajoled, "You've been medicated. You might get dizzy and fall if you sit."

As if I've never been been dizzy before, I thought. I would not buckle. "I'm honestly capable of knowing when I'm dizzy. I'm an adult and am here for a simple procedure. I don't want to be treated like an invalid."

I had to win this battle. I feared that if she made me bend to being treated like a patient, I would become one. I had to convince her that my reason for being there was inconsequential. If she believed me, then it would be true.

She paused and then suggested, "Why don't I roll up the head of your bed and prop you up with pillows?" I agreed to this compromise and signed the truce agreement.

I hummed choruses as nurses and technicians bustled by, stopping at the door to check the work schedule posted beside it. Some carried surgical equipment and some carried coffee cups. Occasionally a pair of eyelids were lifted. As our eyes met, the person would smile, almost shyly, at this chance intimacy in this impersonal world, this land of the living dead. I huddled shivering under the thin sheet and watched. The nurse's eyes noticed mine and then lowered to my shoulders where the sheet was tucked in tightly. Without a word she disappeared and returned in several minutes with a warmed blanket that she tucked next to my skin.

"Thank you," was all I could think of to say. I was warmed as much by her gentle smile as by the blanket.

I was wheeled at last into the operating room where I was met by Dr. Coulter dressed in his rolled pants and moonboot shoes. I slid onto the cold slab and extended my hand to an anesthetist who began immediately to attach my arm.

"I don't have to count backward, do I?" I did not hear her answer.

* * *

"As I suspected, it was just cellulitis—a localized inflammation —absolutely benign."

I woke, instantly clearheaded. My body refused to remain dormant. Bandages were the only evidence of my time asleep.

My former resolve stirred once more too. My purpose in life, to reach out to others, had sustained me for a year after surgery. It must sustain me once again. My illness had equipped me with even more ability to empathize with people's pain. I must shake my worry about whether I would be healthy again. Just as Dad had been useful in illness, I had to be once more. "All things work together for good to them that love God." *I love him. I must allow him to work in my life.*

"You have forgotten God your Savior; you have not remembered the Rock, your fortress."

"I'm listening, Father." I vowed that this time I would always remember that "This is the day which the Lord hath made; we will rejoice . . . in it."

I *would* remember today. And when discouraged, I'd remember God's care for me in the past and know his love never changes. I began immediately to put my resolution into action. I lifted my eyes and prayed, "Oh, Father, it has been a long time, I know, but I just wanted to tell you that I'm still grateful for peristalsis."

*   *   *

Renae and Neil ran to me and tangled their arms around me. Renae acted as spokesman. "We were afraid you wouldn't come home."

"But I told you the infection just needed to be let out. The doctor had to put a drain in my arm under this bandage so that the pus can drain out."

"But I was still afraid," Neil confessed. "I don't like you to go to the hospital."

I looked deeply into my children's eyes. Their faces mirrored my former fears about my own dad. I knew that for Renae and Neil a nagging doubt would remain no matter how much I reassured them with my current good health.

I had to acknowledge that someday I might have to inform the children that I did have another malignancy.

I pulled them to me again and turned my face toward heaven. Silently I prayed, "Help Rex and me to teach these little ones to live each moment until that time—and through that time."

Postscript

THE TREE IN THE FOREST, SHELTERED BY NEIGHBORING TREES, is weak and vulnerable alone. If other trees are removed, a strong wind will destroy it.

The tree in the middle of the yard, bearing the buffets from all angles, is strong. The stress of the storms strengthens it.

I am kin to both these trees: I am protected from the winds by the love of my heavenly Father, my family, my friends. Yet in the solitude of cancer's yard, I am forced to stand tall to face its harsh winds. As the winds die to a breeze, I find I am stronger to face other storms of life.

* * *

Cancer is not the one-word summary of a life; it is not the essence. Life itself is central. The quality of life is what is important—not the means of death.

My grandmother lived a normal life span but died in purpose when she got cancer. Dad lived fewer years but cherished each moment. Ron lost his sense of purpose and tossed away his future. Kris, blocked from faith in her ability to achieve goals or find happiness, has never begun to live.

* * *

A curious student asks me to describe chemotherapy and radiation. I hesitate. "It's like a living hell, isn't it?" he bursts out.

I want to be honest. "Some people would say yes. But what's important is that it is life. And I love living!"

* * *

Most of the time I remind myself that cancer is not the worst disaster.

I recall the Boyer family's catastrophic loss when their son and brother fell from a hay wagon and was run over by a passing car. Still I see the shock lines on the faces of his parents and three sisters. I remember watching the Johnsons' helplessness as they struggled to prevent the suffering of their three-year-old son who had leukemia. And I have seen the agony of a family when a teenager storms out in rebellion or continues to live physically in the house but leaves emotionally—through drugs, alcohol, destructive friends. I know that the pain of losing a child is much sharper than that caused by personal suffering.

Mental pain is much more devastating than physical pain: the agony of splintered relationships through divorce or separation. The aching vacuum of despair after the loss of belief in self and in the future. The anxiety of enduring fears without a sense of purpose, existing in depression and isolation.

A suffering world searches for meaning. Humanity's quest is universal. And I have found the answer; I have found purpose in love and service. Some exist lifetimes and never find a reason for the next breath; I have heard our Father whisper, "Peace I give unto you. Not as the world gives, give I." In the midst of the gales, his serenity calms me.

* * *

But other times I concentrate on the storm and not the peace in the eye of it. I no longer dwell on the "things that are lovely." My childhood lesson that cancer is never really over goads me. I see my tall, bronzed, farmer father shrink to the bleached skeletal cancer patient. Instead of the "still small voice" I hear the chemotherapist's flat statement that there is no cure for cancer; doctors are only investigators. Therefore, I am the guinea pig. My fear is not paranoia: cancer still ranks as the reigning killer. My chemotherapist, who holds hope for a future cure, never takes cancer lightly. When I joke that an excuse from jury duty is a "fringe benefit of cancer," he seriously argues, "There are no benefits of cancer." Scrupulously the doctor catalogs even a minor symptom. "We are a team against a dangerous and unpredictable enemy," he declares. "We need every weapon available to fight this enemy. We must never waste energy fighting each other." Cancer's power is acknowledged and respected.

* * *

But today I am alive, I remind myself. I am thankful for this day's opportunities, I chant.

* * *

"Bill is so sick. He looks so tired and weak."

"You must realize that radiation is debilitating," I encourage his friend. "It'll be months after he has finished his treatments before he'll feel better. But see how much stronger I am now."

"I'll tell him what you said. It will relieve some of his depression."

Two weeks pass. "Bill died."

Slap—my emotions sting.

* * *

Laurie smiles. "Anna is doing so much better. The therapy is really working."

"That's terrific news. Michael is lucky to have such a spunky mother. She was right to defy the doctors and get pregnant."

Laurie walks into our kitchen. Her pale face is streaked. "Anna just died."

"How? What happened? She was doing so much better." I want to scream.

"She was changing Michael's diaper and had a cerebral hemorrhage, I guess."

Slap.

* * *

My friend Marcia drives me to Youngstown for my treatment. We discuss my techniques for tolerating chemotherapy.

"My aunt has so much trouble with nausea."

"I really believe food, even though it gags me, in the long run makes me feel better. I think forced eating and forced activity pays off."

Several months pass. Again she chauffeurs me. "You never mention your aunt any more. Did she try eating to control the nausea?"

Marcia hesitates, shifting her eyes. "I didn't want to tell you. She died last month. That's why Mother went down to Florida."

Slap.

* * *

After a ten-year battle with cancer, I was sure Lois Nichols had beaten it.

"Did you hear? Lois has come home."

"Why?"

"She has come home to die."

Wicked, vicious rumor, I think.

I overhear a sorrowful remark. "Her family couldn't stand to see her. She weighs thirty-two pounds now, they say."

"That's impossible," I want to scream.

"She lies in a fetal position."

Cruel gossip.

And the next week Lois Nichols's obituary in the local paper.

Slap.

* * *

But each time after the initial wave of panic passes, in the stillness, I hear once more—"Whatsoever things are lovely... think on these things."

* * *

"You look so good. Bless the Lord." The minister shakes his head dramatically.

"Yes, bless the Lord and Mary Kay Cosmetics," I remark flippantly, hiding my inner thoughts.

He steps back, shocked.

Whether or not I look good, we should bless the Lord. Whether I recover or eventually die of cancer, bless the Lord. He loves me just the same.

* * *

My mind rebels and composes a poem:

Death lurks behind a maniac cell
plotting the mass murder of the orderly rulers.

Unaware of my body's plot to sabotage me,
I naively plan for tomorrow.

The enemy sneers. The marauding cells chant, "We divide and you perish." The victims in this bizarre war are not the dead. The victims are the struggling sufferers.

And I cry out, "Oh Father, my mind is the most seditious enemy."

Tranquilly he repeats, "Who of you by worrying can add a single moment..."

"Father, I can't seem to remember."

"I will not leave you as orphans."

* * *

The statistics are misleading. Not all individuals with the disease are "victims"—only those who shrivel up and no longer reach out or remain useful. The others should be listed as "cancer victors," even if the case ends in death. For victory over cancer does not depend on living a normal life span. Victory is living each moment of your life abundantly.

* * *

To my chemotherapist I announce, "You're going to be famous. You will be known as the doctor of Janet Britton."

His twinkling black eyes suddenly become serious. "All I want is for Janet Britton to still be alive when I get famous."

He doesn't understand that cancer may kill me, but never conquer me. As a cancer victor, I live every moment on this earth until God pulls up the stakes of my tent and moves my spirit to a new, more permanent location. My tent needs repairs, but I continue to occupy it in spite of minor inconveniences.

* * *

"You can't end your book discussing death. Your book is a book about life. You aren't supposed to get down just because others die."

"But sometimes I do."

"Your book should have a focus. The reader should see the steady development of your faith."

"But my life is not a straight line of growth. I'm not a character in fiction."

"But you have learned what it is to be God's child."

"Yes, I'm positive I'm God's child. But I act like a child, too. Sometimes pouting and irritable. Sometimes obedient and cuddly and unselfish. I guess I have both the strength and the frailties of a child."

My learning is a process, a cyclical pattern. Like Paul, I'm striving and pressing on. But I'll never arrive at perfection on this earth.

* * *

No, cancer is never really over. We are never the same as before. But I'm learning that not being the same is not necessarily terrible, for cancer is one of those things that "kills the body but not the soul." It is not to be feared.

The presence of cancer is just a reminder that we are mortal. We have limited time. We have not a moment to waste on "I should haves" and "what ifs." Therefore we must concentrate on each moment of life. Stop to see the ant shouldering its bundle. Hug and be hugged. Concentrate on our impact on our children. And strive to pass our values on to our children. The threat of recurrence buffets the family as well as the patient. But both can be stronger for it.

The formerly brusque Rex, in a Sunday-school class discussing how to deal with people who are suffering if you aren't, peeped out of a crack in the wall of his castle. Leaving himself vulnerable to the arrows of criticism, he said, "I just wanted to say that I don't think people can be sensitive to other people's suffering until someone they love has been hurting. When you go through someone's hurt, you get more sensitive."

Rex, Renae and Neil are gentle, sensitive people.

* * *

"Who will finish your book after you . . . ?" Rex can't finish his question.

"Die?"

"Well, yes. It's about your life, isn't it? People will want to know how it ends."

"My book is just about a section of my life—when I was on treatment."

"But people won't know what happens to you."

"Oh, yes, they will. They'll know I learned to live every day I had. And I did that with relish. They just won't know if that life was sixty more days or sixty more years. Or if I died of cancer or of being bitten by an asp while on a vacation in Turkey. But that part isn't really important. I lived a full and purposeful life. Besides, ultimately all of us die.

* * *

I remain as long as my Father has work for me to do.